Urology Research Progress

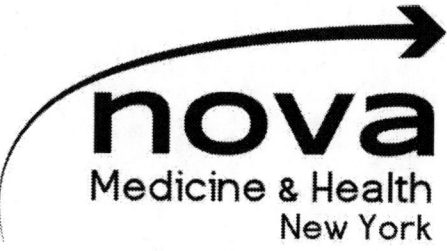

Urology Research Progress

Renal Replacement Therapy: Controversies and Future Trends
José A. Moura-Neto, MD (Editor)
2018. ISBN: 978-1-53613-654-8 (Hardcover)
2018. ISBN: 978-1-53613-655-5 (eBook)

Innovations in Dialysis Vascular Access Surgery
Archil B. Chkhotua (Editor)
2017. ISBN: 978-1-53612-158-2 (Hardcover)
2017. ISBN: 978-1-53612-182-7 (eBook)

Urinary Incontinence: Prevalence, Risk Factors and Management Strategies
Debra Newton (Editor)
2016. ISBN: 978-1-53610-099-0 (Softcover)
2016. ISBN: 978-1-53610-113-3 (eBook)

International Book of Erectile Dysfunction
Miroslav L. Djordjevic, M.D., Ph.D. (Editor)
Francisko E. Martins, M.D. (Editor)
2016. ISBN: 978-1-63485-271-5 (Hardcover)
2016. ISBN: 978-1-63485-289-0 (eBook)

More information about this series can be found at
https://novapublishers.com/product-category/series/urology-research-progress/

Garry M. Morones
Editor

Vesicoureteral Reflux

From Diagnosis to Treatment

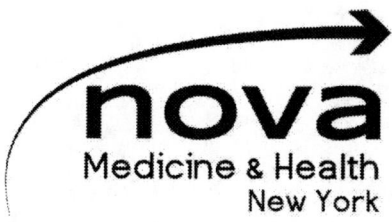

Copyright © 2024 by Nova Science Publishers, Inc.

All rights reserved. No part of this book may be reproduced, stored in a retrieval system or transmitted in any form or by any means: electronic, electrostatic, magnetic, tape, mechanical photocopying, recording or otherwise without the written permission of the Publisher.

We have partnered with Copyright Clearance Center to make it easy for you to obtain permissions to reuse content from this publication. Please visit copyright.com and search by Title, ISBN, or ISSN.

For further questions about using the service on copyright.com, please contact:

Copyright Clearance Center
Phone: +1-(978) 750-8400   Fax: +1-(978) 750-4470   E-mail: info@copyright.com

NOTICE TO THE READER

The Publisher has taken reasonable care in the preparation of this book but makes no expressed or implied warranty of any kind and assumes no responsibility for any errors or omissions. No liability is assumed for incidental or consequential damages in connection with or arising out of information contained in this book. The Publisher shall not be liable for any special, consequential, or exemplary damages resulting, in whole or in part, from the readers' use of, or reliance upon, this material. Any parts of this book based on government reports are so indicated and copyright is claimed for those parts to the extent applicable to compilations of such works.

Independent verification should be sought for any data, advice or recommendations contained in this book. In addition, no responsibility is assumed by the Publisher for any injury and/or damage to persons or property arising from any methods, products, instructions, ideas or otherwise contained in this publication.

This publication is designed to provide accurate and authoritative information with regards to the subject matter covered herein. It is sold with the clear understanding that the Publisher is not engaged in rendering legal or any other professional services. If legal or any other expert assistance is required, the services of a competent person should be sought. FROM A DECLARATION OF PARTICIPANTS JOINTLY ADOPTED BY A COMMITTEE OF THE AMERICAN BAR ASSOCIATION AND A COMMITTEE OF PUBLISHERS.

Library of Congress Cataloging-in-Publication Data

Names: Morones, Garry M., editor.
Title: Vesicoureteral reflux : from diagnosis to treatment / editor Garry M. Morones.
Description: New York : Nova Science Publishers, [2024] | Series: Urology research progress | Includes bibliographical references and index. |
Identifiers: LCCN 2024000714 (print) | LCCN 2024000715 (ebook) | ISBN 9798891134447 (paperback) | ISBN 9798891135055 (adobe pdf)
Subjects: LCSH: Vesico-ureteral reflux in children. | Vesico-ureteral reflux in children--Diagnosis. | Vesico-ureteral reflux in children--Treatment.
Classification: LCC RJ476.V4 V47 2024 (print) | LCC RJ476.V4 (ebook) | DDC 618.92/61--dc23/eng/20240125
LC record available at https://lccn.loc.gov/2024000714
LC ebook record available at https://lccn.loc.gov/2024000715

Published by Nova Science Publishers, Inc. † New York

Contents

Preface	....	vii
Chapter 1	**Urinary Extracellular Vesicles: Potential Biomarkers for Vesicoureteral Reflux**..............1 Cahyani Gita Ambarsari, Chika Carnation Tandri and Gerhard Reinaldi Situmorang	
Chapter 2	**Standards for the Diagnostics and Treatment of Vesicoureteral Reflux in Children in the Russian Federation** ....33 Sergei Nikitin, Natalia Guseva, Svetlana Kononova and Vadim Nikitin	
Chapter 3	**When Does Vesicoureteral Reflux Develop in Children Operated on for a Spinal Hernia?** ....51 Sergei Nikitin, Natalia Guseva, Svetlana Kononova and Vadim Nikitin	
Chapter 4	**Vesicoureteral Reflux in a Child with Combined Pelvic Organ Dysfunction: A Clinical Observation**...67 Sergei Nikitin, Natalia Guseva, Svetlana Kononova and Vadim Nikitin	
Chapter 5	**A Clinical Observation of the Conservative Treatment of Vesicoureteral Reflux on the Background of Detrusor-Sphincter Dyssinergia in an 8-Year-Old Child**..............................83 Sergei Nikitin, Natalia Guseva, Svetlana Kononova and Vadim Nikitin	

Chapter 6	**Neurological Disorders and the Formation of Vesicoureteral Reflux in Children Operated on for Anorectal Malformations .... 95** Sergei Nikitin, Natalia Guseva, Svetlana Kononova and Vadim Nikitin	
Index	.... **111**	

Preface

Six chapters on Vesicoureteral Reflux are included in this book. The first chapter explores the potential of uEVs as noninvasive biomarkers for diagnosing VUR, monitoring its progression, and determining the extent of kidney damage. Chapter Two investigates the Russian Federation's diagnostic and treatment requirements for vesicoureteral reflux in children. Chapter Three goes on to discuss the treatment regimens for spinal neurogenic bladder and its complications – vesicoureteral reflux. The fourth chapter is a clinical observation – the medical history of a 6-year-old girl with combined pelvic organ dysfunction, characterized by hyperactive bladder syndrome and constipation. Another clinical case is presented in Chapter 5, this time with an 8-year-old patient suffering from recurrent urinary tract infection. In Chapter Six, a rehabilitation program for the restoration of bladder function and the conservative treatment of vesicoureteral reflux in children who have previously been operated on for anorectal malformations is provided.

Chapter 1

Urinary Extracellular Vesicles: Potential Biomarkers for Vesicoureteral Reflux

Cahyani Gita Ambarsari[1,2,3,4,*]
Chika Carnation Tandri[1]
and Gerhard Reinaldi Situmorang[1,5]

[1]Faculty of Medicine Universitas Indonesia, Jakarta, Indonesia
[2]Department of Child Health, Cipto Mangunkusumo Hospital, Jakarta, Indonesia
[3]University of Nottingham, Nottingham, UK
[4]Medical Technology Cluster, Indonesian Medical Education and Research Institute (IMERI), Faculty of Medicine, Universitas Indonesia, Jakarta, Indonesia
[5]Department of Urology, Cipto Mangunkusumo Hospital, Jakarta, Indonesia

Abstract

Vesicoureteral reflux (VUR) is characterized by the backward flow of urine from the bladder to the upper urinary tract, causing kidney damage if left untreated. However, the current diagnostic method, voiding cystourethrography (VCUG), is invasive, potentially risky, and may cause anxiety, especially for young patients and their caregivers. Urinary extracellular vesicles (uEVs) are small vesicles originating from the renal tubular system that carry lipids, proteins, and RNAs for intercellular communication and regulation. uEVs have emerged as promising human biofluid-derived biomarkers in various kidney diseases. This chapter explores the potential of uEVs as noninvasive biomarkers for diagnosing VUR, monitoring its progression, and determining the extent of kidney damage.

---

[*] Corresponding Author's Email: cahyani.ambarsari@ui.ac.id.

In: Vesicoureteral Reflux
Editor: Garry M. Morones
ISBN: 979-8-89113-444-7
© 2024 Nova Science Publishers, Inc.

Previously, serum inflammatory markers have been identified as factors associated with kidney fibrosis in reflux nephropathy, but these may simply be a reflection of systemic inflammation rather than of a specific condition. Meanwhile, current research on uEVs in VUR remains limited. One study has identified vitronectin, a uEV-derived protein, as a predictor of VUR induced by spinal cord injury (sensitivity = 80%, specificity = 82.9%, area under the curve (AUC) = 0.795). Another study, focusing on pediatric VUR, showed that patients with kidney fibrosis had significantly higher urinary neutrophil gelatinase-associated lipocalin (uNGAL) values than those without kidney fibrosis (1.49 ng/mL vs. 0.58 ng/mL, $p < 0.001$). However, apart from kidney fibrosis, uNGAL also increases in the contexts of AKI and pediatric urinary tract infections, indicating that uNGAL is not specific as a single marker for VUR. These findings highlight the importance of identifying biomarkers derived from entities, such as uEVs, that are specific to the urinary system and are not affected by systemic factors

In summary, uEVs offer crucial insights into urinary tract processes and have broad potential for diagnosing, treating, and forecasting kidney and urinary tract diseases, including VUR. Future studies to test their role should encompass larger sample sizes, standardized protocols, and rigorous validation.

Keywords: diagnostic, fibrosis, invasive, kidney damage, urinary tract

Introduction

Extracellular vesicles (EVs) constitute a diverse group of lipid-bilayer membrane-enclosed vesicles released by cells into the extracellular space (Figure 1) [1, 2]. They were first observed in 1983 as small vesicles, released from reticulocytes, that carry transferrin receptors [3]. In 1996, EVs were proved to be biologically functional, leading to an interest in biomarker research [4]. EVs are released by various cell types and can be detected in numerous biological fluids, including blood, urine, saliva, breast milk, and cerebrospinal fluid [2]. Under normal physiological circumstances, EVs primarily eliminate undesirable materials from host cells [1], and they play a crucial role in intercellular communication by transporting genetic materials, proteins, and lipids to recipient cells [1, 2].

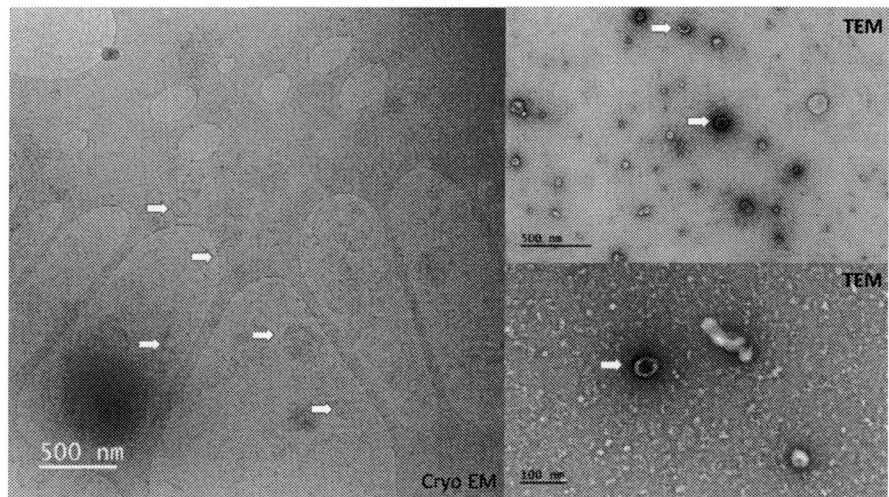

Figure 1. uEVs (white arrow) seen with EM. (a) Cryo-EM characterization of uEVs: single vesicles, double vesicles, double-membrane vesicles, and multilayer vesicles. (b) and (c) TEM characterization of uEVs, uEVs were negatively stained with 2% uranyl acetate.
Cryo-EM: cryogenic electron microscopy; EM: electron microscopy; TEM: transmission electron microscopy; uEVs: urinary extracellular vesicles.

Over the last decade, there has been a surge of interest in the potential of EVs, especially exosomes (the smallest at 20-150 nm), as noninvasive biomarkers and as therapeutic tools [1]. EV-associated molecules, including nucleic acids and proteins, play a part in neoplastic diseases, neurodegenerative conditions, infections, and autoimmune disorders [5–7]. Additionally, EVs have been explored as therapeutic agents [8]. For instance, EVs derived from stem cells or progenitor cells show innate immunosuppressive and anti-inflammatory properties in the treatment of arthritis [9], while modified EVs can serve as vehicles for drug delivery, such as doxorubicin-loaded EVs for the treatment of retinoblastoma [8, 10].

Vesicoureteral reflux (VUR) is the flow of urine backwards from the bladder to the ureters and potentially the kidneys [11]. VUR is often asymptomatic or is discovered during an initial evaluation for urinary tract infections (UTIs), and accounts for 10% of children investigated for their first UTI [12]. However, asymptomatic VUR could lead to delayed detection and potential kidney damage, since 30%–54% of VUR cases had developed kidney parenchymal scarring at diagnosis [12]. Diagnosis of VUR currently relies on voiding cystourethrography (VCUG), which is both invasive and risky [13]. There are also concerns about the accuracy and safety of VCUG, especially during active infections, and the risks of radiation exposure and contrast-related hypersensitivity [13]. Additionally, standard single-phase VCUG may fail to detect intermittent VUR episodes, necessitating a cyclic VCUG involving increased radiation exposure [14]. Furthermore, the reliability of VUR grading through VCUG is questionable, as it relies solely on the observers' judgement. One study demonstrated that only 43% of cases showed agreement between three radiologists [15].

A pilot study comparing urinary proteomes of pediatric VUR patients with those with recurrent UTIs and with normal children found 80 differently expressed proteins [16]. Among these, 62 proteins were associated with UTIs and 18 with kidney injury [16]. However, the urinary proteomes were identified from free urine samples rather than EVs. This chapter elaborates the possible use of urinary EVs (uEVs) in diagnosing VUR, predicting prognosis, assessing the extent of kidney damage and monitoring treatment response.

Extracellular Vesicles: Physiological Roles in Kidneys and Urinary Tract

There are three main groups of EVs: exosomes (20–150 nm), microvesicles (100–1000 nm), and apoptotic bodies (100–5000 nm) (Figure 2) [1, 17]. Other groups are of much smaller size and are known as exopheres or supermeres [18, 19]. There are also larger EVs, such as oncosomes and large renal tubular EVs [18, 19]. These evolving classifications reflect our growing understanding of the diversity and complexity of EVs.

The biogenesis of the three main groups occurs through different pathways (Figure 3). The key distinction between different types of EVs is their specific biogenesis method, which consequently determines their contents and functions. Exosomes originate by inward budding of the cell membrane, forming intracellular endosomes with a reversed membrane topology [18, 20]. These are then sorted into multivesicular bodies (MVBs). When MVBs fuse with the cell membrane, they release the intraluminal vesicles (ILVs) contained within as exosomes. Alternatively, fusion with lysosomes results in degradation [18, 20]. Microvesicles are generated more directly through outward budding of the cell membrane, while apoptotic bodies are generated by extrusion from dying cells. Once released into the extracellular environment, the distinction between exosomes and other EVs becomes challenging due to overlapping content and size, especially in urine [18, 20].

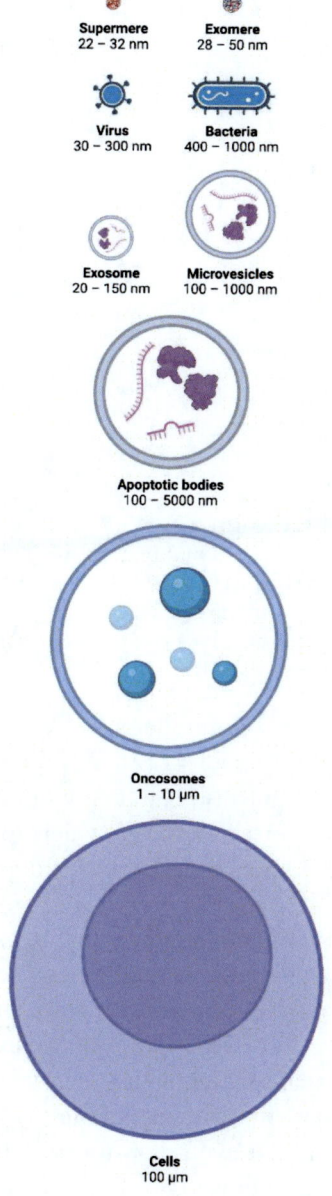

Figure 2. Comparison of extracellular vesicle sizes. Created with BioRender.com.

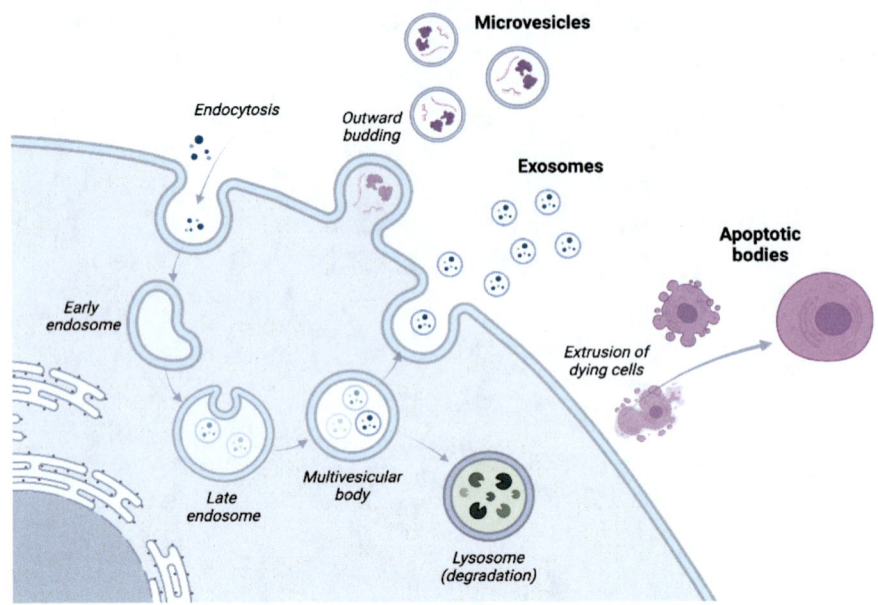

Figure 3. Biogenesis of EVs. Created with BioRender.com.
The cell membrane undergoes inward budding, forming endosomes, which are then converted into multivesicular bodies (MVBs). These MVBs can merge with lysosomes for degradation or with the cell membrane to release exosomes. The outward budding of cell membrane gives rise to microvesicles or apoptotic bodies, for the extrusion of dying cells.

In urine, EVs are derived predominantly from glomerular, tubular, prostate, and bladder cells (Figure 4) [21, 22]. uEVs can also emerge from immune cells and microorganisms [22]. It is worth noting that urine contains a quantity of EVs with a reversed topology, which do not fit into the categories of exosomes, microvesicles, or apoptotic bodies, but instead resemble endosomes [18, 22].

uEVs facilitate intra-nephron communication, spanning both glomerular and tubular regions [23]. The vesicles, released by cells in the upper segments of tubules, can be taken up by downstream cells, thereby transferring active molecules [23, 24]. In this way, EVs contribute to functions such as maintaining cellular balance, regulating electrolytes and water levels, facilitating tubular regeneration, and modulating inflammatory responses [23, 24]. For example, an early study demonstrated that cultured murine kidney collecting duct cells could convey functional aquaporin 2 (AQP2) via the release and uptake of EVs [22, 23]. EVs obtained from proximal tubular cells are absorbed *in vitro* by distal tubule and collecting duct cells [20, 24]. EVs are involved in interactions between the glomerular-tubular, endothelial-podocyte, and tubular-interstitial cell components [25].

EVs play a pivotal role in facilitating long-distance cell-to-cell communication within and outside the kidney and may exacerbate kidney damage [20, 23]. They can amplify inflammation, trigger tubulointerstitial fibrosis, or promote glomerular epithelial-mesenchymal transition (EMT) [23, 27]. Disruption of communication by EVs could compromise podocyte function [20]. Additionally, EVs released by podocytes may facilitate communication between the glomeruli and tubules, potentially promoting tubular injury [26, 27]. This intricate interplay could contribute to increased damage, the development of tubulointerstitial fibrosis, and the progression of chronic kidney disease (CKD) [27].

Under normal conditions, the excretion of uEVs in humans remains relatively constant [1, 2, 18]. However, cellular stress or conditions such as acute kidney injury (AKI) or glomerulonephritis can lead to an increased excretion of uEVs [18]. In a stable state, most uEVs originate from the kidney, since the surface area of nephrons is greater than that of the bladder [20]. A comparison of uEVs from nephrostomy drains and from urine showed nearly identical proteomes [28]. Additionally, the amount of uEVs excreted correlated closely with nephron mass [28]. However, a small percentage of uEVs contain markers not associated with the urogenital system [20]. This only happens in conditions in which the basement membrane is compromised, since an intact glomerular barrier permits the passage only of structures less than 6 nm in size [20, 29].

EVs as Biomarkers of Diseases from All Biofluids

Most research has focused on exosomes, because of their role as intercellular messengers and their potential in disease diagnosis and targeted drug delivery. Whereas the direct budding of cell membranes forms non-exosomal EVs, exosomes originate from the inward budding of endosomes [30]. During this process, exosomes are loaded with specific information in the form of lipids, proteins, and nucleic acids, which can then affect recipient cells without direct cell contact [30].

The most prominent fields of EV research are neoplastic, neurodegenerative, and cardiorespiratory disease. Like healthy cells, tumor cells also release EVs, which can play a role in various aspects of cancer progression, including cell growth, metastasis, angiogenesis and resistance to chemotherapy [31, 32]. Several studies have reported a high sensitivity of serum EVs in detecting cancer, such as miR-1246 for breast cancer and vesicular copine-3 (CPNE3) for colorectal cancer [33, 34]. EV biomarkers have also been established for neurodegenerative diseases, such as α-synuclein in Parkinson's disease and phosphorylated tau proteins (P-T181-tau and P-S396-tau) and amyloid β-protein 1-42 (Aβ1-42) in Alzheimer's disease [35]. EVs have been linked to various cardiovascular disorders, including atherosclerosis, cardiac hypertrophy, myocardial infarction, and heart failure, through several miRNAs, including miR-21, miR-126, and miR-146a [36, 37]. Additionally, EV proteins such as polygenic immunoglobulin receptor (pIgR), cystatin C, and complement factor C5a have been associated with acute coronary syndrome [38]. Bronchial epithelial cell-derived EVs exhibit elevated levels of miR-210 and miR-21 in chronic obstructive pulmonary disease and WNT5A protein in idiopathic lung fibrosis [39]. The role of EVs as disease biomarkers are summarized in Table 1.

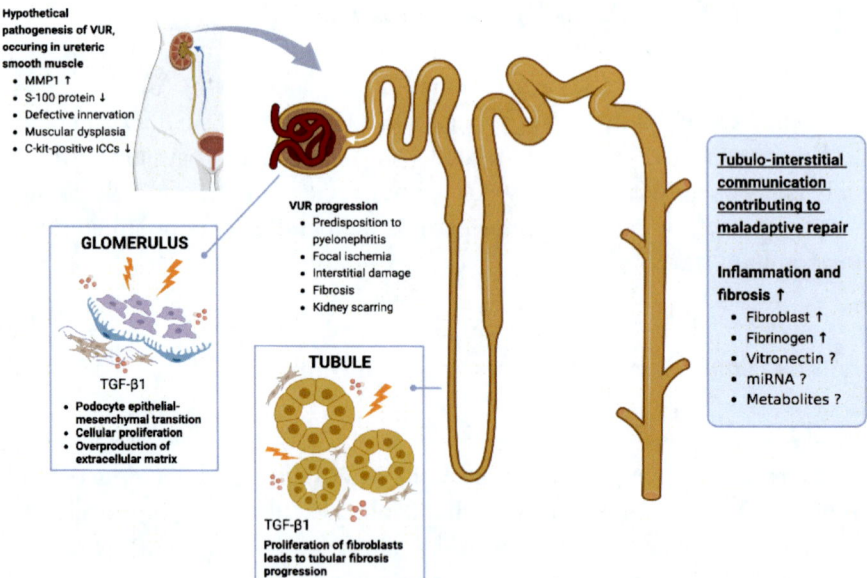

Figure 4. uEVs representing tubular system cells, the role in VUR. Created with BioRender.com.
ICCs: interstitial cells of Cajal; miRNA: micro-ribonucleic acid; MMP1: matrix metalloproteinase 1; TGF-β1: transforming growth factor-β1; uEVs: urinary extracellular vesicles; VUR: vesicoureteral reflux.

Table 1. EVs as disease biomarkers

Diseases	Biomarker Type	Source	Specific Biomarkers	Biomarker performance	References
Breast cancer	miRNA	Serum	miR-1246	Upregulated	Li 2017 [33]
Colorectal cancer	RNA	Serum	CPNE3	Upregulated	Sun 2019 [34]
Parkinson's disease	Protein	Plasma, cerebrospinal fluid	α-synuclein	Upregulated	Stuendl 2016, [40] Shi 2014, [41] Cao 2019 [42]
Alzheimer's disease	Protein	Plasma	P-T181-tau, P-S396-tau, Aβ1-42	Upregulated	Fiandaca 2015,[43] Winston 2016 [44]
Atherosclerotic cardiovascular disease	miRNA	Plasma	miR-21, miR-126, miR-146a	Upregulated	Das 2015 [36]
Acute coronary syndrome	Protein	Plasma	pIgR, cystatin C, and C5a	Upregulated	De Hoog 2013 [38]
Chronic obstructive pulmonary disease	miRNA	Broncho-alveolar lavage fluid	miR-210, miR-21	Upregulated	Fujita 2015, [45] Xu 2018 [46]
Idiopathic lung fibrosis	Protein	Broncho-alveolar lavage fluid	WNT5A	Upregulated	Martin-Medina 2018 [47]

CPNE3: copine-3; P-T181-tau: phosphorylated tau proteins-T181; P-S396-tau: phosphorylated tau protein-S396; Aβ1-42: amyloid β-protein 1-42; pIgR: polygenic immunoglobulin receptor; C5a: complement factor 5a; WNT5A: Wingless-related integration site (Wnt) family member 5A

Table 2. Research on EVs as diagnostic biomarkers in kidney diseases

Diseases	Type	Source	Biomarkers	Biomarker performance	References
Prostate cancer	RNA	Urine	PCA3, ERG	Upregulated	Nilsson 2009, [52] Donovan 2015 [53]
	miRNA	Urine, serum, plasma, semen	miR-21, miR-574, miR-375, miR-141, miR-142	Upregulated	Li Z 2015, [54] Li W 2020, [55] Barcelo 2019 [56]
Polycystic kidney disease	Protein	Urine	Periplakin, envoplakin, villin-1	Upregulated	Salih 2016 [57]
Diabetic nephropathy	Protein	Urine	WT1	Upregulated	Abe 2018 [58]
	Protein	Urine	AMBP, MLL3, and VDAC1	Upregulated	Zubiri 2014 [59]
Acute kidney injury	Protein	Urine	AQP1	Downregulated	Sonoda 2009 [60]
Glomerulonephritis	Protein	Urine	Acute crescentic: FSP1	Upregulated	Morikawa 2019 [61]
Chronic kidney disease	miRNA	Urine	miR-29c	Downregulated	Chun-Yan 2018 [62]
Lupus nephritis	miRNA	Urine	miR-21, let-7a	Downregulated	Tangtanatakul 2019 [63]
Tubulopathies	Protein	Urine	Gitelman syndrome: NCC	Downregulated	Corbetta 2015, [64] Williams 2020 [65]
	Protein	Urine	Bartter syndrome: NKCC2	Downregulated	Corbetta 2015 [64]
	Protein	Urine	Salt-losing tubulopathies (Gitelman & Bartter): TSG101, FLOT1, VPS4A, VPS4B, AQP2, DPEP1, CA2, ANXA7, ANXA11	Upregulated	Raimondo 2020 [66]

Diseases	Type	Source	Biomarkers	Biomarker performance	References
Hypertension	Protein	Urine	Hypertension with albuminuria: OLFM4, AT3, MPO	Increased: OLFM4, AT3 Decreased: MPO	Gonzalez-Calero 2017 [67]
	Protein	Urine	Renovascular hypertension: nephrin, podocalyxin	Upregulated	Kwon 2017 [68]
	Protein	Urine	NCC, ENaC	Upregulated	Qi 2016 [69]
	Protein	Urine	Hypertension with cushing syndrome: pNKCC2, pNCC	Upregulated	Salih 2016 [70]
	Protein	Urine	Primary aldosteronism: NCC, pNCC	Upregulated	Wolley 2017, [71] van der Lubbe 2012 [72]

PCA3: prostate cancer antigen 3; ERG: erythroblast transformation-specific-related gene; miR: microRNA; WT1: Wilms tumor 1; AMBP: alpha-1-microglobulin/bikunin precursor; MLL3: mixed-lineage leukemia protein 3; VDAC1: voltage-dependent anion-selective channel 1; AQP1: aquaporin 1; FSP1: ferroptosis suppressor protein 1; NCC: sodium-chloride cotransporter; NKCC2: sodium-potassium-2 chloride cotransporter; TSG101: tumor susceptibility gene 101; FLOT1: flotillin-1; VPS4A: vacuolar protein sorting-associated protein 4A; VPS4B: vacuolar protein sorting-associated protein 4B; AQP2: aquaporin 2; DPEP1: dipeptidase 1; CA2: carbonic anhydrase 2; ANXA7: annexin A7; ANXA11: annexin A11; OLFM4: olfactomedin 4; AT3: antithrombin 3; MPO: myeloperoxidase; ENaC: epithelial sodium channel; pNKCC2: phosphorylated sodium-potassium-2 chloride cotransporter; pNCC: phosphorylated sodium-chloride cotransporter

EVs as Kidney Biomarkers

Since 2012, following recommendations from the Kidney Disease Improving Global Outcomes (KDIGO), work on non-invasive biomarkers has continued [48]. This is crucial, since standard assessments using spot urine evaluations can sometimes be conflicting [49, 50]. Outcome assessment is also crucial since kidney diseases have the tendency to damage multiple organs, especially the cardiovascular system [51].

Early work focused on neoplasms of the urogenital system, leading to the discovery of biomarkers such as proteins, mRNA, miRNA, lipids, and metabolites for prostate, bladder and renal cancers [20]. Two prostate cancer-related RNAs, prostate cancer antigen 3 (PCA3) and transmembrane protease serine 2:v-ets erythroblastosis virus E26 oncogene homolog (TMPRSS2:ERG), were validated in two prospective multi-center studies in the United States [21]. These results led to further work on the potential use of uEV-based biomarkers in other kidney and urogenital tract pathologies, including polycystic kidney disease (PKD), diabetic nephropathy, AKI, CKD, glomerulonephritis, lupus nephritis, and tubulopathies, as well as primary and secondary hypertension (Table 2).

EVs as Therapeutic Agents or Carriers in Various Kidney Diseases

EVs play an integral role in intercellular communication, both within the kidney and with other organs. Cultured cell-derived EVs may also exhibit therapeutic potential. EVs can serve as therapeutic agents either by acting as carriers for drugs and nucleic acids or by making use of their natural content [48]. Suitable cells include activated antigen-presenting cells (APC), natural killer cells, mesenchymal stem cells (MSC), and endothelial progenitor cells (EPCs) [73]. Furthermore, EVs derived from tumors carry and transmit tumor antigens to APCs, fostering anti-tumor responses.

EVs have demonstrated potential as drug delivery systems due to their small size, exceptional permeability, minimal immunogenicity, and non-cytotoxic nature. The small size of exosomes allows evasion of rapid clearance by mononuclear phagocytes [74]. Zhuang et al. [76] have shown that uEVs in the form of exosomes delivered intranasally can pass the blood brain barrier and allow rapid delivery of anti-inflammatory drugs to the brain.

Using uEVs as therapeutic agents requires a 'loading' process, which can be divided into pre-loading (before isolation) and post-loading (after isolation). Pre-loading methods involve loading drugs into uEVs during cell growth. Post-loading involves loading drugs into isolated uEVs. The methods used in pre- and post-loading techniques are similar, consisting of incubation, infection and the use of ultrasound combined with microbubbles. Successful drug loading into uEVs has been achieved with various agents, including curcumin, hyaluronic acid, and b-blocker carvedilol. All have shown good stability and sustained therapeutic function [77].

MSCs possess a unique capacity for kidney repair through their anti-fibrotic effects, although MSC-associated tumorigenic effects and MSC rejection have been reported [78, 79]. EVs do not have a cellular structure: they are not tumorigenic and have low immunogenicity [78, 80]. Moreover, EVs from MSCs mimic the immunomodulatory and cytoprotective functions of the original cells. Administration of MSC-derived EVs can restore kidney structure and function in various experimental models of AKI [73]. MSC-derived EVs can protect the kidney by modulating the immune response, preventing apoptosis, and stimulating cell proliferation. Many molecules may be involved, including miR-let7c, known for its anti-fibrotic properties; interleukin 10 (IL-10), which exhibits anti-inflammatory properties, and miR-126 and miR-296, which promote the regeneration of kidney cells [73, 81–84]. Other miRNAs have also been reported to affect cell infiltration, proliferation, epithelial-mesenchymal transition, and apoptosis inhibition in tubular epithelial cells and endothelial cells [85, 86].

A prior study explored the impact of human umbilical cord mesangial stem cell-derived exosomes (hucMSC-Exos) on a mouse model with kidney injury induced by VUR rising from partial bladder outlet obstruction. The intravenous administration of hucMSC-Exos, proved effective in reducing the expression of proteins linked to the Wnt/β-catenin signaling pathway [87]. This led to the inhibition of cellular proliferation and the reversal of kidney damage. These findings underscore the potential of EVs as a novel therapeutic approach for addressing VUR.

In addition to serving as therapeutic agents, EVs can also serve as biomarkers, aiding in monitoring therapeutic responses by capturing specific molecular states. Recent emerging evidence has substantiated the pivotal roles of EVs in driving cancer progression and metastasis, highlighting their substantial potential in therapeutic applications [88]. A prospective open-label and blinded endpoint (PROBE) crossover study by Pathare et al. has highlighted the use of EVs as biomarkers of a particular therapy [89]. The study showed that the abundance of Na-Cl Cotransporter (NCC) was correlated with the reduction of blood pressure induced by hydrochlorothiazide (HCT). It was found that unprocessed NCC is processed into uEVs after complex glycosylation steps [89].

Pathogenesis and Pathophysiology of Vesicoureteral Reflux

Primary VUR is associated with a congenital abnormality of the vesicoureteral junction (VUJ) [90]. The VUJ serves as the boundary between the low pressure of the upper urinary tract and the higher pressure of the lower urinary tract. It protects the upper tract against reflux by employing active and passive anti-reflux mechanisms. The active mechanism involves the contraction of the longitudinal muscle layers in the transmural and submucosal regions of the ureter, pushing urine into the bladder, while the passive mechanism involves the compression of the upper portion of the intravesical ureter against the underlying detrusor muscle. Any functional or structural changes, including short intravesical ureter length and large ureteral orifice diameter, may disrupt the closure of the VUJ, leading to VUR [90]. In contrast, secondary VUR occurs without apparent abnormality of the VUJ. Instead, it is due to an increase in intravesical pressure usually associated with bladder outlet obstruction, voiding dysfunction, or neurologic abnormalities [90].

Abnormalities in smooth muscle cells and innervation are associated with VUR (Figure 4) [90, 91]. Impaired innervation of the distal ureteral endings alters the active anti-reflux mechanism. Increased expression of matrix metalloproteinase 1 (MMP1) in CD68+ cells has also been reported [85, 86]. Additionally, a marker for innervation in the ureteral wall, S-100 protein, was significantly reduced in neural cells of refluxing ureters [90]. Muscle dysplasia, atrophy, and cell irregularities have been reported in patients with refluxing ureters [92]. This dysplasia is characterized by a reduction and disruption in smooth muscle bundles, leading to uncoordinated muscular contractions and the loss of c-kit-positive interstitial cells of Cajal (ICCs), responsible for pacemaker activity at the VUJ level [93, 90].

If undetected and left untreated, VUR may cause further damage to the upper urinary tract, particularly the kidneys. VUR can potentially contribute to the development of CKD and end-stage kidney disease [94–98]. The backflow of the urine causes an increase in intratubular hydrostatic pressure, with tubular ischemia, mechanical stretching or compression of tubular cells and changes in urinary shear stress [99]. These are associated with the dysregulation of various cytokines, growth factors, enzymes, and cytoskeletal proteins. Initial alterations in kidney hemodynamics are followed by structural and functional changes across the nephron referred to as reflux nephropathy (RN) [99]. The degree of VUR is classified using a grading system (I to V) based on the observations made during VCUG. Ureter dilatation and other anatomical abnormalities are marked between grade III and grade V, with one study reporting that 71% of patients with grade III to V had GFR <40% of expected, while 18% experienced kidney deterioration [100].

In the earliest stage of VUR, there is a 1–2 hour increase in renal blood flow. Subsequently, the intrarenal renin–angiotensin–aldosterone system is activated, resulting in vasoconstriction in pre- and post-glomerular areas, with decreased renal blood flow, medullary oxygen tension, and glomerular filtration rate. The increased angiotensin II within the kidney activates nuclear factor kappa B, triggering the release of cytokines and the production of reactive oxygen species (ROS). Adhesion molecules, including selectins, attract macrophages to the area, upregulate monocyte chemotactic protein-1 (MCP-1), and release tumor necrosis factor-α (TNF-α). Monocytes and macrophages migrate to the tubular interstitium in the obstructed kidney. Activated macrophages infiltrate the interstitium, perpetuating inflammation by releasing cytokines such as transforming growth factor-β1 (TGF-β1), TNF-α, and ROS. ROS mediates the profibrotic effects of TGF-β1, leading to interstitial fibrosis characterized by increased extracellular matrix deposition, cellular infiltration, tubular apoptosis, and EMT. Mild injury triggers apoptosis, while severe injury may lead to necrosis. Increased apoptosis and/or necrosis activate cell infiltration, interstitial cell proliferation, and interstitial fibrosis. Eventually, these processes lead to the development of fibrotic tissue in the kidney parenchyma [99, 101].

Various cytokines and chemokines, including TGF-β, IL-10, IL-6, IL-8, and TNF, play a significant role in VUR and the formation of RN. Elevated levels of IL-8/CXCL8 have been observed in the urine of patients with VUR and renal scars. At the same time, increased expression of C-C motif ligand 2/monocyte chemotactic protein-1 (CCL2/MCP-1) can lead to the release of proinflammatory and profibrotic cytokines. Furthermore, IL-6 levels in serum and urine of young children with acute febrile pyelonephritis are correlated with future renal scarring. Elevated TNF levels have been detected in patients with RN, and urinary and serum levels of TGF-β have been associated with renal scarring in VUR. Polymorphisms in the gene encoding IL-10 have also been linked to an increased risk of VUR [101, 102].

Growth factors such as vascular endothelial growth factor (VEGF) and fibroblast growth factor (FGF) have also been associated with early-stage VUR and RN development. Serum levels of vascular cell adhesion molecule

1 (VCAM-1) are significantly increased in patients with high-grade VUR, regardless of the presence of renal scarring, while intercellular adhesion molecule 1 (ICAM-1) may contribute to renal damage. Procalcitonin levels in serum have also been associated with high-grade VUR and RN. The utilization of serum for biomarkers requires care, since they can be influenced by general systemic factors, including inflammation, and more specific biomarkers are needed [102].

Urinary EVs as Biomarkers in VUR

Few studies have explored the use of uEVs as biomarkers in VUR. Li et al. analyzed biomarkers from urinary exosomes in spinal cord injury-induced VUR in adult patients [103]. Damage to the spinal cord may lead to neurogenic bladder, which can elevate detrusor pressure. The urine exosomes were isolated, and their proteomic profile was analyzed by mass spectrometry (MS). This showed 134 upregulated and 99 downregulated protein expressions in the VUR group compared to the non-VUR group. Based on analysis of the peak of peptide segments, 18 candidate proteins were selected for parallel reaction monitoring (PRM) validation. Only vitronectin and α-1 type I collagen (COL1A1) showed significant differences. Enzyme-linked immunosorbent assay (ELISA) results further suggested that urinary exosomal vitronectin could distinguish and predict VUR in patients with neurogenic bladder with a sensitivity of 80%, a specificity of 82.9%, and area under the receiver operating characteristic (ROC) curve (AUC) of 0.795 (95% confidence interval (CI), 0.667–0.923) [103].

An earlier study involving patients with kidney transplantation (KT) reported that uEV vitronectin was found to be a significant marker for chronic interstitial and tubular lesions [104]. KT patients were classified on clinical parameters and graft biopsy as normal kidney function (NKF), interstitial fibrosis and tubular atrophy (IFTA), calcineurin inhibitors toxicity (CNIT) and acute cellular rejection (ACR). Among 23 uEV proteins identified by MS as having differential expression among the four groups, targeted proteomics demonstrated a differential expression of vitronectin in patients with graft biopsies showing ci and ct mean > 2 according to Banff criteria. These results were further validated with ELISA (AUC 0.87) [104].

Urine exosomal vitronectin can originate from either the kidney or the bladder. Recent research on urine exosomal vitronectin has indicated a positive correlation with kidney fibrosis [104]. Additionally, Li et al. proposed that exosomal vitronectin is linked to fibrosis in the neurogenic bladder [103]. The primary pathological factors hypothesized to contribute to decreased bladder compliance are bladder remodelling and fibrosis, leading to urine reflux and kidney damage [103].

Additionally, genetic associations to VUR have been reported. Genetic loci on chromosome 1p13 and 2q37 under autosomal dominant inheritance have been found in patients with primary VUR, with linkage among siblings [105]. The American Urological Association (AUA) reported that the incidence of VUR in siblings of children with VUR is approximately 27% [106]. Therefore, uEV-associated genetic materials hold promise as diagnostic indicators.

Future Perspectives

The use of uEVs as biomarkers for diagnosis, prognosis, and guidance for treatment, as well in treatment itself, poses many challenges. There are gaps in methodology and knowledge that need to be overcome. These include fundamental laboratory methods like urine collection, uEV separation and measurement, and normalization, to ensure robustness, reliability, credibility, and sustainability [21].

A position paper from the International Society of Extracellular Vesicles (ISEV) has mentioned a lack of rigor and standardization in uEV study protocols [21]. Potential artifacts and contaminants, including microbiota, must be identified. Because urine is one of the most dynamic biofluids, the development of urine collection and storage protocols, along with standard operating procedures, will enhance the reliability and reproducibility of uEV studies [21]. Databases should be created to better understand the impact of variables using the pre-analytical information from multiple studies. One of these is the EV-TRACK platform [107].

EV-TRACK is an online toolset developed by ISEV to improve transparency in reporting and centralizing knowledge in EV research. EV-TRACK comprises seven features that consolidate data on EV characteristics and methods of ongoing and published EV studies. At the same time, EV-TRACK coaches researchers in the use of EV-METRIC while the studies are being conducted. Nine experimental parameters currently reported in EV-METRIC comprise six EV characterization-related parameters (EV-enriched proteins, at least one non-EV-enriched protein, antibody specifics, lysate preparation, qualitative and quantitative analysis, and electron microscopy images) and three EV separation-related parameters (density gradient, EV density, and ultracentrifugation specifics). In the future, a further challenge will be to translate findings from laboratory setting into real-world clinical applications [107].

Current work on uEVs as VUR biomarkers is promising, but its credibility will rely on validation within a larger cohort of patients. Because urine collection is minimally invasive and urine can be collected in large quantities, uEVs as biomarkers will enable physicians to monitor VUR patients more frequently, reducing reliance on VCUG and on cyclic VCUG in the case of intermittent VUR. uEVs may be able to identify specific molecular markers and could complement VCUG as the initial standard diagnostic procedure [14, 108, 109]. Furthermore, uEVs will allow earlier diagnosis and delivery of the best treatments to regulate fibrosis and scarring [110]. The outcomes of these studies can shape the long-term kidney health of VUR patients and enhance their overall quality of life.

While there has been limited direct research on uEVs in VUR, valuable lessons can be drawn from investigations into biomarkers in other kidney conditions. Despite focusing on different diseases and not using uEVs, several notable papers offer methodological and analytical considerations that may be adaptable to the study of uEVs in VUR [111, 112].

A systematic review of urinary Neutrophil Gelatinase-Associated Lipocalin (uNGAL) in VUR management in children provides a significant foundation for the topics of urine biomarkers in VUR [111]. uNGAL has been suggested as an early predictor for kidney damage in diseases such as AKI, UTI, and various CKD causes such as nephrotic syndrome, type 1 diabetes, and urinary tract malformations, including VUR [113–115]. Naik et al. concluded that uNGAL can serve as a biomarker for renal scars in pediatric VUR. Children with VUR with kidney fibrosis had higher median uNGAL levels than those without (1.49 ng/mL vs. 0.58 ng/mL, $p < 0.001$) [115]. However, uNGAL's sensitivity and specificity in detecting VUR-associated kidney fibrosis were both limited to 71% (AUC = 0.769) [116].

Conflicting results regarding the correlation between uNGAL levels and renal scarring and between uNGAL levels and the presence of VUR and VUR grading have been reported [111, 116]. Furthermore, the sensitivity and specificity of uNGAL for small children are lower because of insufficient renal tubular cells with the residual regenerative capacity to produce high levels of uNGAL [117]. Therefore, uNGAL cannot replace VCUG in the diagnosis of VUR, although it might be useful in assessing the indications for surgery and may render imaging studies unnecessary [118]. One important point to consider is that uNGAL levels also increase in the context of AKI and UTI. Hence, the reliability of uNGAL alone as a biomarker for primary VUR in children is not appropriate [111].

There are also concerns regarding the need for urinary creatinine adjustment to the uNGAL levels, which may vary with other factors such as water intake, time of sample collection, hydration status, and urine output [111, 119]. Issues regarding the clinical validation of reagents also raises questions about their analytical performance and reliability [120]. These facts underscore the importance of identifying biomarkers originating from urinary tract cells that remain unaffected by factors external to the urinary system [111]. While uNGAL has yet to be established as a biomarker for VUR, the approach in evaluating uNGAL as a biomarker emphasises the importance of meticulously assessment of candidate molecules in uEVs.

The future use of uEVs in the treatment of VUR holds great promise. The field of VUR treatment could benefit from other innovations that enhance the therapeutic approach and minimize the need for invasive procedures. Currently, endoscopic injection of bulking agents is recommended as a first-line therapy for the majority of VUR cases, with shorter hospital stays, a low incidence of complications, and a high success rate [121, 122].

The possible use of EVs as a delivery system for VUR treatment is intriguing, since EVs are stable and well-suited for targeted therapy [76, 77]. However, surgical management may be inevitable for severe cases of VUR. Surgical ureteral reimplantation is indicated for patients not responding to endoscopic injection, those diagnosed with grade V VUR, recurrent pyelonephritis, persistent reflux, and other anatomical defects such as refluxing megaureter [11, 122]. In this context, uEV biomarkers might benefit post-surgical monitoring. Long-term monitoring of VCUG assessments following endoscopic or surgical treatment is recommended by the AUA Guidelines 2017 [106], in spite of associated risks and radiation exposure [122]. Both endoscopic injection and surgical reimplantation carry the risk of complications, including the possibility of obstruction due to stenosis or kinking [11]. uEVs could improve the management of VUR by offering a less invasive and potentially more effective treatment while circumventing the need for invasive post-surgical monitoring methods.

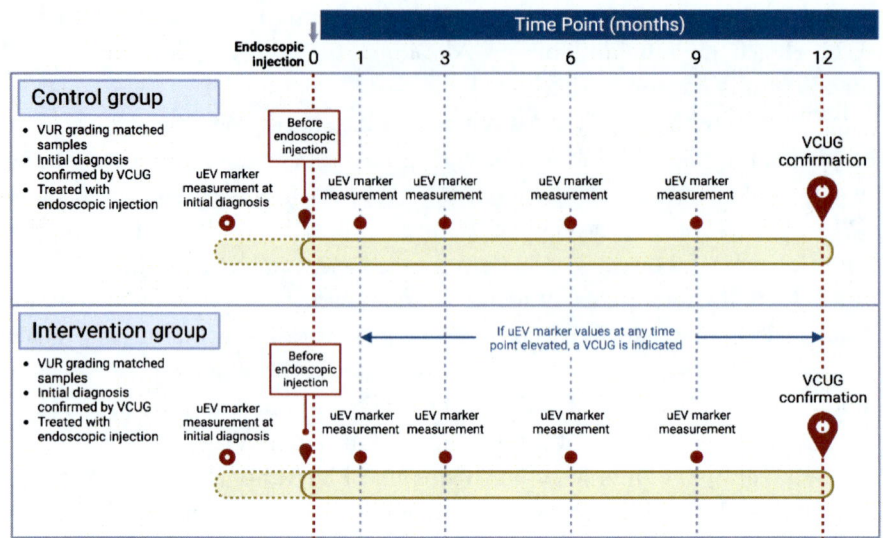

Figure 5. Potential study design of uEV research in post-intervention VUR monitoring. Created with BioRender.com.
uEV: urinary extracellular vesicles; VCUG: voiding cystourethrography; VUR: vesicoureteral reflux.

Another notable paper describing the role of urine noninvasive biomarker in kidney problems investigates urinary chemokine CXCL10 in kidney transplantation monitoring to detect graft rejection [111]. This is crucial, since 27.3% of patients experience graft failure and need to return to dialysis [123, 124]. Two groups, an intervention group and a control group, underwent urine CXCL10 level monitoring at 1, 3, and 6 months after transplantation. Two consecutive urine CXCL10 analyses at the three time points (weeks 4 and 5, weeks 10 and 11, and weeks 22 and 24) defined the differences in the management between the two groups. In the intervention group, a kidney graft biopsy was indicated if CXCL10 values increased in the absence of confounders (UTI and BK polyoma virus replication), followed by subsequent therapy based on the biopsy results. Conversely, urine CXCL10 results remained concealed until the end of the study in the control group. Although the clinical or subclinical rejection incidence, based on Banff 2015 and 2019, was numerically higher in the intervention arm, this study did not demonstrate a beneficial effect of urine CXCL10 monitoring after 1 year, with graft loss and rejection as the primary outcomes and interstitial fibrosis/tubular atrophy, proteinuria, and immunosuppression-related complications as the secondary outcomes [112].

While the CXCL10 study was not directly related to uEVs in VUR, it exemplifies a robust methodology for monitoring post-surgical outcomes using a specific urinary biomarker. As the field of uEVs continues to evolve, drawing inspiration from such studies can enhance our understanding of how uEV biomarkers might be employed to monitor and manage VUR in post-intervention settings. In designing future uEV trials, a combination of longitudinal biomarker measurements, targeted interventions triggered by biomarker thresholds, and comprehensive outcome assessments may serve as a valuable blueprint for future research (Figure 5) [112].

Conclusion

In conclusion, uEVs represent a crucial resource, giving specific insights into the molecular processes, physiological conditions, and pathological states within the urinary tract. EVs possess broad utility in diagnosing, treating, and forecasting outcomes for various diseases, including those that impact the kidney and urinary tract. An uEV-based biomarker is particularly necessary for VUR, since the current diagnostic approach, which involves the invasive and risk-prone VCUG procedure, calls for a more child-friendly alternative. While research on uEVs in VUR remains limited, with only vitronectin studied extensively, valuable insights can be gained from comparable investigations into biomarkers for other kidney conditions. Future studies should focus on multi-center or larger sample sizes, adherence to standardized protocols and sufficient validation procedures, to ensure that uEVs can play a more prominent role in the diagnosis and management of VUR.

References

[1] Doyle, L. M., and Wang, M. Z. (2019). Overview of extracellular vesicles, their origin, composition, purpose, and methods for exosome isolation and analysis. *Cells.*, 8(7), 727. doi: 10.3390/cells8070727.

[2] Di Bella, M. A. (2022). Overview and update on extracellular vesicles: Considerations on exosomes and their application in modern medicine. *Biology (Basel).*, 11(6), 804. doi: 10.3390/biology11060804.

[3] Harding, C., Heuser, J., and Stahl, P. (1983). Receptor-mediated endocytosis of transferrin and recycling of the transferrin receptor in rat reticulocytes. *J Cell Biol.*, 97(2), 329–39. doi: 10.1083/jcb.97.2.329.

[4] Pisitkun, T., Shen, R. F., and Knepper, M. A. (2004). Identification and proteomic profiling of exosomes in human urine. *Proc Natl Acad Sci USA.*, 101(36), 13368–73. doi: 10.1073/pnas.0403453101.

[5] Ciferri, M. C., Quarto, R., and Tasso, R. (2021). Extracellular vesicles as biomarkers and therapeutic tools: from pre-clinical to clinical applications. *Biology (Basel).*, 10(5), 359. Doi: 10.3390/biology10050359.

[6] Lak, N. S. M., van der Kooi, E. J., Enciso-Martinez, A., Lozano-Andrés, E., Otto C., Wauben, M. H. M., and Tytgat, G. A. M. (2022). Extracellular vesicles: A new source of biomarkers in pediatric solid tumors? A systematic review. *Front Oncol.*, 12, 887210. doi: 10.3389/fonc.2022.887210.

[7] Raghav, A., Singh, M., Jeong, G. B., Giri, R., Agarwal, S., Kala, S., and Gautam, K. A. (2022). Extracellular vesicles in neurodegenerative diseases: A systematic review. *Front Mol Neurosci.*, 15, 1061076. doi: 10.3389/fnmol.2022.1061076.

[8] Du, S., Guan, Y., Xie, A., Yan, Z., Gao, S., Li, W., Rao, L., Chen, X., and Chen, T. (2023). Extracellular vesicles: A rising star for therapeutics and drug delivery. *J Nanobiotechnology.*, 21(1), 231. doi: 10.1186/s12951-023-01973-5.

[9] Cosenza, S., Toupet, K., Maumus, M., Luz-Crawford, P., Blanc-Brude, O., Jorgensen, C., and Noël, D. (2018). Mesenchymal stem cells-derived exosomes are more immunosuppressive than microparticles in inflammatory arthritis. *Theranostics.*, 8(5), 1399–410. doi: 10.7150/thno.21072.

[10] Farhat, W., Yeung, V., Kahale, F., Parekh, M., Cortinas, J., Chen, L., Ross, A. E., and Ciolino, J. B. (2022). Doxorubicin-loaded extracellular vesicles enhance tumor cell death in retinoblastoma. *Bioengineering (Basel).*, 9(11), 671. doi: 10.3390/bioengineering9110671.

[11] Blais, A. S., Bolduc, S., and Moore, K. (2017). Vesicoureteral reflux: from prophylaxis to surgery. *Can Urol Assoc J.*, 11(1-2Suppl1), S13–8. doi: 10.5489/cuaj.4342.

[12] Chang, J. W., Liu, C. S., and Tsai, H. L. (2022). Vesicoureteral reflux in children with urinary tract infections in the inpatient setting in Taiwan. *Clin Epidemiol.*, 14, 299–307. doi: 10.2147/CLEP.S346645.

[13] Johnin, K., Kobayashi, K., Tsuru, T., Yoshida, T., Kageyama, S., and Kawauchi, A. (2019). Pediatric voiding cystourethrography: An essential examination for urologists but a terrible experience for children. *Int J Urol.*, 26(2), 160–71. doi: 10.1111/iju.13881.

[14] Papadopoulou, F., Efremidis, S. C., Oiconomou, A., Badouraki, M., Panteleli, M., Papachristou, F., and Soteriou, I. (2002). Cyclic voiding cystourethrography: is vesicoureteral reflux missed with standard voiding cystourethrography? *Eur Radiol.*, 12(3), 666–70. doi: 10.1007/s003300101108.

[15] Schaeffer, A. J., Greenfield, S. P., Ivanova, A., Cui, G., Zerin, J. M., Chow, J. S., et al. (2017). Reliability of grading of vesicoureteral reflux and other findings on voiding cystourethrography. *J Pediatr Urol.*, 13(2), 192–8. doi: 10.1016/j.jpurol.2016.06.020.

[16] Vitko, D., Cho, P. S., Kostel, S. A., DiMartino, S. E., Cabour, L. D., Migliozzi, M. A., Logvinenko, T., Warren, P. G., Froehlich, J. W., and Lee, R. S. (2020). Characterizing patients with recurrent urinary tract infections in vesicoureteral

reflux: A pilot study of the urinary proteome. *Mol Cell Proteomics.*, 19(3), 456–66. doi: 10.1074/mcp.RA119.001873.

[17] Cricrì, G., Bellucci, L., Montini, G., and Collino, F. (2021). Urinary extracellular vesicles: Uncovering the basis of the pathological processes in kidney-related diseases. *Int J Mol Sci.*, 22(12), 6507. doi: 10.3390/ijms22126507.

[18] Erdbrügger, U., Hoorn, E. J., Le, T. H., Blijdorp, C. J., and Burger, D. (2023). Extracellular vesicles in kidney diseases: Moving forward. *Kidney360.*, 4(2), 245–57. doi: 10.34067/KID.0001892022.

[19] Jeppesen, D. K., Zhang, Q., Franklin, J. L., and Coffey, R. J. (2023). Extracellular vesicles and nanoparticles: Emerging complexities. *Trends Cell Biol.*, 33(8), 667–81. doi: 10.1016/j.tcb.2023.01.002.

[20] Grange, C., and Bussolati, B. (2022). Extracellular vesicles in kidney disease. *Nat Rev Nephrol.*, 18(8), 499–513. doi: 10.1038/s41581-022-00586-9.

[21] Erdbrügger, U., Blijdorp, C. J., Bijnsdorp, I. V., Borràs, F. E., Burger, D., Bussolati, B., et al. (2021). Urinary extracellular vesicles: A position paper by the Urine Task Force of the International Society for Extracellular Vesicles. *J Extracell Vesicles.*, 10(7), e12093. Doi: 10.1002/jev2.12093.

[22] Svenningsen, P., Sabaratnam, R., and Jensen, B. L. (2020). Urinary extracellular vesicles: Origin, role as intercellular messengers and biomarkers; efficient sorting and potential treatment options. *Acta Physiol (Oxf).*, 228(1), e13346. Doi: 10.1111/apha.13346.

[23] Lee, S. A., Choi, C., and Yoo, T. H. (2021). Extracellular vesicles in kidneys and their clinical potential in renal diseases. *Kidney Res Clin Pract.*, 40(2), 194–207. doi: 10.23876/j.krcp.20.209.

[24] Kwon, S. H. (2019). Extracellular vesicles in renal physiology and clinical applications for renal disease. *Korean J Intern Med.*, 34(3), 470–9. doi: 10.3904/kjim.2019.108.

[25] van Niel, G., D'Angelo, G., and Raposo, G. (2018). Shedding light on the cell biology of extracellular vesicles. *Nat Rev Mol Cell Biol.*, 19(4), 213–28. doi: 10.1038/nrm.2017.125.

[26] Kosanović, M., Milutinovic, B., Glamočlija, S., Morlans, I. M., Ortiz, A., and Bozic, M. (2022). Extracellular vesicles and acute kidney injury: Potential therapeutic avenue for renal repair and regeneration. *Int J Mol Sci.*, 23(7), 3792. doi: 10.3390/ijms23073792.

[27] Delrue, C., De Bruyne, S., Speeckaert, R., and Speeckaert, M. M. (2023). Urinary extracellular vesicles in chronic kidney disease: from bench to bedside? *Diagnostics (Basel).*, 13(3), 443. doi: 10.3390/diagnostics13030443.

[28] Blijdorp, C. J., Hartjes, T. A., Wei, K. Y., van Heugten, M. H., Bovée, D. M., Budde, R. P. J., et al. (2022). Nephron mass determines the excretion rate of urinary extracellular vesicles. *J Extracell Vesicles.*, 11(1), e12181. doi: 10.1002/jev2.12181.

[29] Huang, J., Brenna, C., Khan, A. M., Daniele, C., Rudolf, R., Heuveline, V., and Gretz, N. (2019). A cationic near infrared fluorescent agent and ethyl-cinnamate tissue clearing protocol for vascular staining and imaging. *Sci Rep.*, 9(1), 521. doi: 10.1038/s41598-018-36741-1.

[30] Li, X., Corbett, A. L., Taatizadeh, E., Tasnim, N., Little, J. P., Garnis, C., Daugaard, M., Guns, E., Hoorfar, M., and Li, I. T. S. (2019). Challenges and opportunities in exosome research-Perspectives from biology, engineering, and cancer therapy. *APL Bioeng.*, 3(1), 011503. doi: 10.1063/1.5087122.

[31] Irmer, B., Chandrabalan, S., Maas, L., Bleckmann, A., and Menck, K. (2023). Extracellular vesicles in liquid biopsies as biomarkers for solid tumors. *Cancers (Basel).*, 15(4), 1307. doi: 10.3390/cancers15041307.

[32] Chang, W. H., Cerione, R. A., and Antonyak, M. A. (2021). Extracellular vesicles and their roles in cancer progression. *Methods Mol Biol.*, 2174, 143–70. doi: 10.1007/978-1-0716-0759-6_10.

[33] Li, X. J., Ren, Z. J., Tang, J. H., and Yu, Q. (2017). Exosomal microRNA miR-1246 promotes cell proliferation, invasion and drug resistance by targeting CCNG2 in breast cancer. *Cell Physiol Biochem.*, 44(5), 1741–8. doi: 10.1159/000485780.

[34] Sun, B., Li, Y., Zhou, Y., Ng, T. K., Zhao, C., Gan, Q., Gu, X., and Xiang, J. (2019). Circulating exosomal CPNE3 as a diagnostic and prognostic biomarker for colorectal cancer. *J Cell Physiol.*, 234(2), 1416–25. doi: 10.1002/jcp.26936.

[35] Yuan, Q., Li, X. D., Zhang, S. M., Wang, H. W., and Wang, Y. L. (2019). Extracellular vesicles in neurodegenerative diseases: Insights and new perspectives. *Genes Dis.*, 8(2), 124–32. doi: 10.1016/j.gendis.2019.12.001.

[36] Das, S., and Halushka, M. K. (2015). Extracellular vesicle microRNA transfer in cardiovascular disease. *Cardiovasc Pathol.*, 24(4), 199–206. doi: 10.1016/j.carpath.2015.04.007.

[37] Chong, S. Y., Lee, C. K., Huang, C., Ou, Y. H., Charles, C. J., Richards A. M., et al. (2019). Extracellular vesicles in cardiovascular diseases: Alternative biomarker sources, therapeutic agents, and drug delivery carriers. *Int J Mol Sci.*, 20(13), 3272–…. doi: 10.3390/ijms20133272.

[38] de Hoog, V. C., Timmers, L., Schoneveld, A. H., Wang, J. W., van de Weg, S. M., Sze, S. K., et al. (2013). Serum extracellular vesicle protein levels are associated with acute coronary syndrome. *Eur Heart J Acute Cardiovasc Care.*, 2(1), 53–60. doi: 10.1177/2048872612471212.

[39] Holtzman, J., and Lee, H. (2020). Emerging role of extracellular vesicles in the respiratory system. *Exp Mol Med.*, 52(6), 887–95. doi: 10.1038/s12276-020-0450-9.

[40] Stuendl, A., Kunadt, M., Kruse, N., Bartels, C., Moebius, W., Danzer, K. M., Mollenhauer, B., and Schneider, A. (2016). Induction of α-synuclein aggregate formation by CSF exosomes from patients with Parkinson's disease and dementia with Lewy bodies. *Brain.*, 139(Pt 2), 481–94. doi: 10.1093/brain/awv346.

[41] Shi, M., Liu, C., Cook, T. J., Bullock, K. M., Zhao, Y., Ginghina, C., et al. (2014). Plasma exosomal α-synuclein is likely CNS-derived and increased in Parkinson's disease. *Acta Neuropathol.*, 128(5), 639–50. doi: 10.1007/s00401-014-1314-y.

[42] Cao, Z., Wu, Y., Liu, G., Jiang, Y., Wang, X., Wang, Z., and Feng, T. (2019). α-Synuclein in salivary extracellular vesicles as a potential biomarker of Parkinson's disease. *Neurosci Lett.*, 696, 114–20. doi: 10.1016/j.neulet.2018.12.030.

[43] Fiandaca, M. S., Kapogiannis, D., Mapstone, M., Boxer, A., Eitan, E., Schwartz J. B., et al. (2015). Identification of preclinical Alzheimer's disease by a profile of

pathogenic proteins in neurally derived blood exosomes: A case-control study. *Alzheimers Dement.*, 11(6), 600–7.e1. doi: 10.1016/j.jalz.2014.06.008.

[44] Winston, C. N., Goetzl, E. J., Akers, J. C., Carter, B. S., Rockenstein, E. M., Galasko, D., Masliah, E., and Rissman, R. A. (2016). Prediction of conversion from mild cognitive impairment to dementia with neuronally derived blood exosome protein profile. *Alzheimers Dement (Amst).*, 3, 63–72. doi: 10.1016/j.dadm.2016.04.001.

[45] Fujita, Y., Araya, J., Ito, S., Kobayashi, K., Kosaka, N., Yoshioka, Y., Kadota, T., Hara, H., Kuwano, K., and Ochiya, T. (2015). Suppression of autophagy by extracellular vesicles promotes myofibroblast differentiation in COPD pathogenesis. *J Extracell Vesicles.*, 4, 28388. doi: 10.3402/jev.v4.28388.

[46] Xu, H., Ling, M., Xue, J., Dai, X., Sun, Q., Chen, C., et al. (2018). Exosomal microRNA-21 derived from bronchial epithelial cells is involved in aberrant epithelium-fibroblast cross-talk in COPD induced by cigarette smoking. Theranostics., 8(19), 5419–33. doi: 10.7150/thno.27876.

[47] Martin-Medina, A., Lehmann, M., Burgy, O., Hermann, S., Baarsma, H. A., Wagner, D. E., et al. (2018). Increased extracellular vesicles mediate WNT5A signaling in idiopathic pulmonary fibrosis. *Am J Respir Crit Care Med.*, 198(12), 1527–38. doi: 10.1164/rccm.201708-1580OC.

[48] Kidney Disease: Improving Global Outcomes (KDIGO) Glomerular Diseases Work Group. KDIGO clinical practice guideline for acute kidney injury. *Kidney Int Suppl.*, 2012, 2, 1–138.

[49] Ambarsari, C. G., Utami, D. A. P., Tandri, C. C., and Satari, H. I. (2023). Comparison of three spot proteinuria measurements for pediatric nephrotic syndrome: based on the International Pediatric Nephrology Association 2022 Guidelines. *Ren Fail.*, 45(2), 2253324. doi: 10.1080/0886022X.2023.2253324.

[50] Ambarsari, C. G., Tambunan, T., Pardede, S. O., Fazlur, Rahman, F. H., and Kadaristiana, A. (2021). Role of dipstick albuminuria in progression of paediatric chronic kidney disease. *J Pak Med Assoc.*, 71(Suppl 2)(2), S103–6.

[51] Palupi-Baroto, R., Hermawan, K., Murni, I. K., Nurlitasari, T., Prihastuti, Y., Sekali, D. R. K., and Ambarsari, C. G. (2021). High fibroblast growth factor 23 as a biomarker for severe cardiac impairment in children with chronic kidney disease: a single tertiary center study. *Int J Nephrol Renovasc Dis.*, 14, 165–71. doi: 10.2147/IJNRD.S304143.

[52] Nilsson, J., Skog, J., Nordstrand, A., Baranov, V., Mincheva-Nilsson, L., Breakefield, X. O., and Widmark, A. (2009). Prostate cancer-derived urine exosomes: A novel approach to biomarkers for prostate cancer. *Br J Cancer.*, 100(10), 1603–7. doi: 10.1038/sj.bjc.6605058.

[53] Donovan, M. J., Noerholm, M., Bentink, S., Belzer, S., Skog, J., O'Neill, V., Cochran, J. S., and Brown, G. A. (2015). A molecular signature of PCA3 and ERG exosomal RNA from non-DRE urine is predictive of initial prostate biopsy result. *Prostate Cancer Prostatic Dis.*, 18(4), 370–5. doi: 10.1038/pcan.2015.40.

[54] Hao, X. K., Li, Z., Ma, Y. Y., Wang, J., Zeng, X. F., Li, R., and Kang, W. (2015). Exosomal microRNA-141 is upregulated in the serum of prostate cancer patients. *Onco Targets Ther.*, 9, 139–48. doi: 10.2147/OTT.S95565.

[55] Li, W., Dong, Y., Wang, K. J., Deng, Z., Zhang, W., and Shen, H. F. (2020). Plasma exosomal miR-125a-5p and miR-141-5p as non-invasive biomarkers for prostate cancer. *Neoplasma.*, 67(6), 1314–8. doi: 10.4149/neo_2020_191130N1234.

[56] Barceló, M., Castells, M., Bassas, L., Vigués, F., and Larriba, S. (2019). Semen miRNAs contained in exosomes as non-invasive biomarkers for prostate cancer diagnosis. *Sci Rep.*, 9(1), 13772. doi: 10.1038/s41598-019-50172-6.

[57] Salih, M., Demmers, J. A., Bezstarosti, K., Leonhard, W. N., Losekoot, M., van Kooten, C., et al. (2016). Proteomics of urinary vesicles links plakins and complement to polycystic kidney disease. *J Am Soc Nephrol.*, 27(10), 3079–92. doi: 10.1681/ASN.2015090994.

[58] Abe, H., Sakurai, A., Ono, H., Hayashi, S., Yoshimoto, S., Ochi, A., et al. (2018.). Urinary exosomal mRNA of WT1 as diagnostic and prognostic biomarker for diabetic nephropathy. *J Med Invest.*, 65(3.4), 208–15. doi: 10.2152/jmi.65.208.

[59] Zubiri, I., Posada-Ayala, M., Sanz-Maroto, A., Calvo, E., Martin-Lorenzo, M., Gonzalez-Calero, L., et al. (2014). Diabetic nephropathy induces changes in the proteome of human urinary exosomes as revealed by label-free comparative analysis. *J Proteomics.*, 96, 92–102. doi: 10.1016/j.jprot.2013.10.037.

[60] Sonoda, H., Yokota-Ikeda, N., Oshikawa, S., Kanno, Y., Yoshinaga, K., Uchida, K., et al. (2009). Decreased abundance of urinary exosomal aquaporin-1 in renal ischemia-reperfusion injury. *Am J Physiol Renal Physiol.*, 297(4), F1006-16. doi: 10.1152/ajprenal.00200.2009.

[61] Morikawa, Y., Takahashi, N., Kamiyama, K., Nishimori, K., Nishikawa, Y., Morita, S., et al. (2019). Elevated levels of urinary extracellular vesicle fibroblast-specific protein 1 in patients with active crescentic glomerulonephritis. *Nephron.*, 141(3), 177–87. doi: 10.1159/000495217.

[62] Chun-Yan, L., Zi-Yi, Z., Tian-Lin, Y., Yi-Li, W., Bao, L., Jiao, L., and Wei-jun, D. (2018). Liquid biopsy biomarkers of renal interstitial fibrosis based on urinary exosome. *Exp Mol Pathol.*, 105(2), 223–8. doi: 10.1016/j.yexmp.2018.08.004.

[63] Tangtanatakul, P., Klinchanhom, S., Sodsai, P., Sutichet, T., Promjeen, C., Avihingsanon, Y., and Hirankarn, N. (2019). Down-regulation of let-7a and miR-21 in urine exosomes from lupus nephritis patients during disease flare. *Asian Pac J Allergy Immunol.*, 37(4), 189–97. doi: 10.12932/AP-130318-0280.

[64] Corbetta, S., Raimondo, F., Tedeschi, S., Syrèn, M. L., Rebora, P., Savoia, A., Baldi, L., Bettinelli, A., and Pitto, M. (2015). Urinary exosomes in the diagnosis of Gitelman and Bartter syndromes. *Nephrol Dial Transplant.*, 30(4), 621–30. doi: 10.1093/ndt/gfu362.

[65] Williams, T. L., Bastos, C., Faria, N., Karet, and Frankl, F. E. (2020). Making urinary extracellular vesicles a clinically tractable source of biomarkers for inherited tubulopathies using a small volume precipitation method: proof of concept. *J Nephrol.*, 33(2), 383–6. doi: 10.1007/s40620-019-00653-8.

[66] Raimondo, F., Chinello, C., Porcaro, L., Magni, F., and Pitto, M. (2020). Urinary extracellular vesicles and salt-losing tubulopathies: A proteomic approach. *Proteomes.*, 8(2), 9. doi: 10.3390/proteomes8020009.

[67] Gonzalez-Calero, L., Martínez, P. J., Martin-Lorenzo, M., Baldan-Martin, M., Ruiz-Hurtado, G., de la Cuesta, F., et al. (2017). Urinary exosomes reveal protein

signatures in hypertensive patients with albuminuria. *Oncotarget.*, 8(27), 44217–31. doi: 10.18632/oncotarget.17787.
[68] Kwon, S. H., Woollard, J. R., Saad, A., Garovic, V. D., Zand, L., Jordan, K. L., Textor, S. C., and Lerman, L. O. (2017). Elevated urinary podocyte-derived extracellular microvesicles in renovascular hypertensive patients. *Nephrol Dial Transplant.*, 32(5), 800–7. doi: 10.1093/ndt/gfw077.
[69] Qi, Y., Wang, X., Rose, K. L., MacDonald, W. H., Zhang, B., Schey, K. L., and Luther, J. M. (2016). Activation of the endogenous renin-angiotensin-aldosterone system or aldosterone administration increases urinary exosomal sodium channel excretion. *J Am Soc Nephrol.*, 27(2), 646–56. doi: 10.1681/ASN.2014111137.
[70] Salih, M., Bovée, D. M., van der Lubbe, N., Danser, A. H. J., Zietse, R., Feelders, R. A., and Hoorn, E. J. (2018). Increased urinary extracellular vesicle sodium transporters in cushing syndrome with hypertension. *J Clin Endocrinol Metab.*, 103(7), 2583–91. doi: 10.1210/jc.2018-00065.
[71] Wolley, M. J., Wu, A., Xu, S., Gordon, R. D., Fenton, R. A., and Stowasser M. (2017). In primary aldosteronism, mineralocorticoids influence exosomal sodium-chloride cotransporter abundance. *J Am Soc Nephrol.*, 28(1), 56–63. doi: 10.1681/ASN.2015111221.
[72] van der Lubbe, N., Jansen, P. M., Salih, M., Fenton, R. A., van den Meiracker, A. H., Danser, A. H., Zietse, R., and Hoorn, E. J. (2012). The phosphorylated sodium chloride cotransporter in urinary exosomes is superior to prostasin as a marker for aldosteronism. *Hypertension.*, 60(3), 741–8. doi: 10.1161/HYPERTENSIONAHA.112.198135.
[73] Lv, L. L., Wu, W. J., Feng, Y., Li, Z. L., Tang, T. T., and Liu, B. C. (2018). Therapeutic application of extracellular vesicles in kidney disease: Promises and challenges. *J Cell Mol Med.*, 22(2), 728–37. doi: 10.1111/jcmm.13407.
[74] Klyachko, N. L., Arzt, C. J., Li, S. M., Gololobova, O. A., and Batrakova, E. V. (2020). Extracellular vesicle-based therapeutics: Preclinical and clinical investigations. *Pharmaceutics.*, 12(12), 1171. doi: 10.3390/pharmaceutics12121171.
[75] Han, Y., Jones, T. W., Dutta, S., Zhu, Y., Wang, X., Narayanan, S. P., Fagan, S. C., and Zhang, D. (2021). Overview and update on methods for cargo loading into extracellular vesicles. *Processes (Basel).*, 9(2), 356. doi: 10.3390/pr9020356.
[76] Zhuang, X., Xiang, X., Grizzle, W., Sun, D., Zhang, S., Axtell, R. C., et al. (2011). Treatment of brain inflammatory diseases by delivering exosome encapsulated anti-inflammatory drugs from the nasal region to the brain. *Mol Ther.*, 19(10), 1769–79. doi: 10.1038/mt.2011.164.
[77] Du, S., Guan, Y., Xie, A., Yan, Z., Gao, S., Li, W., Rao, L., Chen, X., and Chen, T. (2023). Extracellular vesicles: A rising star for therapeutics and drug delivery. *J Nanobiotechnology.*, 21(1), 231. doi:10.1186/s12951-023-01973-5.
[78] Caldas, H. C., Lojudice, F. H., Dias, C., Fernandes-Charpiot, I. M. M., Baptista, M. A. S. F., Kawasaki-Oyama, R. S., Sogayar, M. C., Takiya, C. M., and Abbud-Filho, M. (2017). Induced pluripotent stem cells reduce progression of experimental chronic kidney disease but develop Wilms' tumors. *Stem Cells Int.*, 2017, 7428316. doi: 10.1155/2017/7428316.

[79] Koch, M., Lehnhardt, A., Hu, X., Brunswig-Spickenheier, B., Stolk, M., Bröcker, V., Noriega, M., Seifert, M., and Lange, C. (2013). Isogeneic MSC application in a rat model of acute renal allograft rejection modulates immune response but does not prolong allograft survival. *Transpl Immunol.*, 29(1-4), 43-50. doi: 10.1016/j.trim.2013.08.004.

[80] Lou, G., Chen, Z., Zheng, M., and Liu, Y. (2017). Mesenchymal stem cell-derived exosomes as a new therapeutic strategy for liver diseases. *Exp Mol Med.*, 49(6), e346. doi: 10.1038/emm.2017.63.

[81] Wang, B., Yao, K., Huuskes, B. M., Shen, H. H., Zhuang, J., Godson, C., Brennan, E. P., Wilkinson-Berka, J. L., Wise, A. F., and Ricardo, S. D. (2016). Mesenchymal stem cells deliver exogenous microRNA-let7c via exosomes to attenuate renal fibrosis. *Mol Ther.*, 24(7), 1290–301. doi: 10.1038/mt.2016.90.

[82] Eirin, A., Zhu, X. Y., Puranik, A. S., Tang, H., McGurren, K. A., van Wijnen, A. J., Lerman, A., and Lerman, L. O. (2017). Mesenchymal stem cell-derived extracellular vesicles attenuate kidney inflammation. *Kidney Int.*, 92(1), 114–24. doi: 10.1016/j.kint.2016.12.023.

[83] Barile, L., and Vassalli, G. (2017). Exosomes: Therapy delivery tools and biomarkers of diseases. *Pharmacol Ther.*, 174, 63–78. doi: 10.1016/j.pharmthera.2017.02.020.

[84] Cantaluppi, V., Gatti, S., Medica, D., Figliolini, F., Bruno, S., Deregibus, M. C., Sordi, A., Biancone, L., Tetta, C., and Camussi, G. (2012). Microvesicles derived from endothelial progenitor cells protect the kidney from ischemia-reperfusion injury by microRNA-dependent reprogramming of resident renal cells. *Kidney Int.*, 82(4), 412–27. doi: 10.1038/ki.2012.105.

[85] Merchant, M. L., Rood, I. M., Deegens, J. K. J., and Klein, J. B. (2017). Isolation and characterization of urinary extracellular vesicles: Implications for biomarker discovery. *Nat Rev Nephrol.*, 13(12), 731–49. doi:10.1038/nrneph.2017.148.

[86] Zhao, N., Koenig, S. N., Trask, A. J., Lin, C. H., Hans, C. P., Garg, V., and Lilly, B. (2015). MicroRNA miR145 regulates TGFBR2 expression and matrix synthesis in vascular smooth muscle cells. *Circ Res.*, 116(1), 23–34. doi:10.1161/CIRCRESAHA.115.303970.

[87] Wang, Z., Yu, Y., Jin, L., Tan, X., Liu, B., Zhang, Z., et al. (2023). HucMSC exosomes attenuate partial bladder outlet obstruction-induced renal injury and cell proliferation via the Wnt/β-catenin pathway. *Eur J Pharmacol.*, 952, 175523. doi: 10.1016/j.ejphar.2023.175523.

[88] Stevic, I., Buescher, G., and Ricklefs, F. L. (2020). Monitoring therapy efficiency in cancer through extracellular vesicles. *Cells.*, 9(1), 130. doi: 10.3390/cells9010130.

[89] Pathare, G., Tutakhel, O. A. Z., van der Wel, M. C., Shelton, L. M., Deinum, J., Lenders, J. W. M., Hoenderop, J. G. J., and Bindels, R. J. M. (2017). Hydrochlorothiazide treatment increases the abundance of the NaCl cotransporter in urinary extracellular vesicles of essential hypertensive patients. *Am J Physiol Renal Physiol.*, 312(6), F1063–72. doi: 10.1152/ajprenal.00644.2016.

[90] Arena, S., Iacona, R., Impellizzeri, P., Russo, T., Marseglia, L., Gitto, E., and Romeo, C. (2016). Physiopathology of vesico-ureteral reflux. *Ital J Pediatr.*, 42(1), 103. doi: 10.1186/s13052-016-0316-x.

[91] Oswald, J., Schwentner, C., Brenner, E., Deibl, M., Fritsch, H., Bartsch, G., and Radmayr, C. (2004). Extracellular matrix degradation and reduced nerve supply in refluxing ureteral endings. *J Urol.*, 172(3), 1099–102. doi: 10.1097/01.ju.0000135673.28496.70.

[92] Tokunaka, S., Gotoh, T., Koyanagi, T., and Miyabe, N. (1984). Muscle dysplasia in megaureters. *J Urol.*, 131(2), 383–90. doi: 10.1016/s0022-5347(17)50391-2.

[93] Schwentner, C., Oswald, J., Lunacek, A., Fritsch, H., Deibl, M., Bartsch, G., and Radmayr, C. (2005). Loss of interstitial cells of Cajal and gap junction protein connexin 43 at the vesicoureteral junction in children with vesicoureteral reflux. *J Urol.*, 174(5), 1981–6. doi: 10.1097/01.ju.0000176818.71501.93.

[94] Santoso, D. N., Sinuraya, F. A. G., and Ambarsari, C. G. (2022). Distal renal tubular acidosis presenting with an acute hypokalemic paralysis in an older child with severe vesicoureteral reflux and syringomyelia: a case report. *BMC Nephrol.*, 23(1), 248. doi: 10.1186/s12882-022-02874-9.

[95] Wente-Schulz, S., Aksenova, M., Awan, A., Ambarsari, C. G., Becherucci, F., Emma, F., et al. (2021). Aetiology, course and treatment of acute tubulointerstitial nephritis in paediatric patients: a cross-sectional web-based survey. *BMJ Open.*, 11(5), e047059. doi: 10.1136/bmjopen-2020-047059.

[96] Ambarsari, C. G., Trihono, P. P., Kadaristiana, A., Rachmadi, D., Andriastuti, M., Puspitasari, H. A., Tambunan, T., Pardede, S. O., Mangunatmadja, I., and Hidayati, E. L. (2020). Low-dose maintenance intravenous iron therapy can prevent anemia in children with end-stage renal disease undergoing chronic hemodialysis. *Int J Nephrol.*, 2020, 3067453–8. doi: 10.1155/2020/3067453.

[97] Ambarsari, C. G., Hidayati, E. L., Mushahar, L., and Kadaristiana, A. (2020). Dressing versus non-dressing technique for long-term exit-site care in children on continuous ambulatory peritoneal dialysis: a single-center retrospective cohort study. *Med J Indones.*, 29(3), 290–7. doi: 10.13181/mji.oa.204171.

[98] Ambarsari, C. G., Trihono, P. P., Kadaristiana, A., Tambunan, T., Mushahar, L., Puspitasari, H. A., Hidayati, E. L., and Pardede, S. O. (2019). Five-year experience of continuous ambulatory peritoneal dialysis in children: a single center experience in a developing country. *Med J Indones.*, 28(4), 329–37. doi: 10.13181/mji.v28i4.3807.

[99] Washino, S., Hosohata, K., and Miyagawa, T. (2020). Roles played by biomarkers of kidney injury in patients with upper urinary tract obstruction. *Int J Mol Sci.*, 21(15), 5490. doi: 10.3390/ijms21155490.

[100] Sjöström, S., Jodal, U., Sixt, R., Bachelard, M., and Sillén, U. (2009). Longitudinal development of renal damage and renal function in infants with high grade vesicoureteral reflux. *J Urol.*, 181(5), 2277–83. doi: 10.1016/j.juro.2009.01.051.

[101] Colceriu, M. C., Aldea, P. L., Răchişan, A. L., Clichici, S., Sevastre-Berghian, A., and Mocan, T. (2023). Vesicoureteral reflux and innate immune system: Physiology, physiopathology, and clinical aspects. *J Clin Med.*, Mar 19, 12(6), 2380. doi: 10.3390/jcm12062380.

[102] Valério, F. C., Lemos, R. D., de, C., Reis, A. L., Pimenta, L. P., Vieira, É. L., and Silva, A. C. E. (2020). Biomarkers in vesicoureteral reflux: An overview. *Biomark Med.*, 14(8), 683–96. doi: 10.2217/bmm-2019-0378.

[103] Li, J., Cai, S., Zeng, C., Chen, L., Zhao, C., Huang, Y., and Cai, W. (2022). Urinary exosomal vitronectin predicts vesicoureteral reflux in patients with neurogenic bladders and spinal cord injuries. *Exp Ther Med.*, 23(1), 65. doi: 10.3892/etm.2021.10988.

[104] Carreras-Planella, L., Cucchiari, D., Cañas, L., Juega, J., Franquesa, M., Bonet, J., et al. (2021). Urinary vitronectin identifies patients with high levels of fibrosis in kidney grafts. *J Nephrol.*, 34(3), 861–74. doi: 10.1007/s40620-020-00886-y.

[105] Feather, S. A., Malcolm, S., Woolf, A. S., Wright, V., Blaydon, D., Reid, C. J., et al. (2000). Primary, nonsyndromic vesicoureteric reflux and its nephropathy is genetically heterogeneous, with a locus on chromosome 1. *Am J Hum Genet.*, 66(4), 1420–5. doi: 10.1086/302864.

[106] Peters, C. A., Skoog, S. J., Arant, B. S., Jr, Copp, H. L., Elder, J. S., Hudson, R. G., et al. (2017). Management and screening of primary vesicoureteral reflux in children [Internet]. Maryland: American Urological Association; 2017 [cited on 2023 Oct 13]. Available at: https://www.auanet.org/guidelines-and-quality/guidelines/vesicoureteral-reflux-guideline.

[107] Van Deun, J., Mestdagh, P., Agostinis, P., Akay, Ö., Anand, S., Anckaert, J., et al. (2017). EV-TRACK: transparent reporting and centralizing knowledge in extracellular vesicle research. *Nat Methods.*, 14(3), 228–32. doi: 10.1038/nmeth.4185.

[108] Kim, Y. J., Cho, B. S., Lee, J., Ryu, H., Byun, H., Yeon, M., Park, Y., Oh, C., and Jeon, Y. (2020). The ABCs of voiding cystourethrography. *Taehan Yongsang Uihakhoe Chi.*, 81(1), 101–18. doi: 10.3348/jksr.2020.81.1.101.

[109] Arlen, A. M., Amin, J., and Leong, T. (2022). Voiding cystourethrogram: Who gets a cyclic study and does it matter? *J Pediatr Urol.*, 18(3), 378–82. doi: 10.1016/j.jpurol.2022.02.008.

[110] Vanhove, T., Goldschmeding, R., and Kuypers, D. (2017). Kidney fibrosis: Origins and interventions. *transplantation.*, 101(4), 713–26. doi: 10.1097/TP.0000000000001608.

[111] Gavrilovici, C., Dusa, C. P., Iliescu, Halitchi, C., Lupu, V. V., Spoiala, E. L., Bogos, R. A., et al. (2023). The role of urinary NGAL in the management of primary vesicoureteral reflux in children. *Int J Mol Sci.*, 24(9) 7904. doi: 10.3390/ijms24097904.

[112] Hirt-Minkowski, P., Handschin, J., Stampf, S., Hopfer, H., Menter, T., Senn, L., et al. (2023). Randomized trial to assess the clinical utility of renal allograft monitoring by urine CXCL10 chemokine. *J Am Soc Nephrol.*, 34(8), 1456–69. doi: 10.1681/ASN.0000000000000160.

[113] Shyam, R., Patel, M. L., Sachan, R., Kumar, S., and Pushkar, D. K. (2017). Role of urinary neutrophil gelatinase-associated lipocalin as a biomarker of acute kidney injury in patients with circulatory shock. *Indian J Crit Care Med.*, 21(11), 740–45. doi: 10.4103/ijccm.IJCCM_315_17.

[114] Uwaezuoke, S. N., Ayuk, A. C., Muoneke, V. U., and Mbanefo, N. R. (2018). Chronic kidney disease in children: Using novel biomarkers as predictors of disease. *Saudi J Kidney Dis Transpl.*, 29(4), 775–84. doi: 10.4103/1319-2442.239657.

[115] Mamilly, L., Mastrandrea, L. D., Mosquera, Vasquez, C., Klamer, B., Kallash, M., and Aldughiem, A. (2021). Evidence of early diabetic nephropathy in pediatric type 1 diabetes. *Front Endocrinol (Lausanne).*, 12, 669954. doi: 10.3389/fendo.2021.669954.
[116] Naik, P. B., Jindal, B., Kumaravel, S., Halanaik, D., Rajappa, M., Naredi, B. K., and Govindarajan, K. K. (2022). Utility of urinary biomarkers neutrophil gelatinase-associated lipocalin and kidney injury molecule-1 as a marker for diagnosing the presence of renal scar in children with vesicoureteral reflux (VUR): A cross-sectional study. *J Indian Assoc Pediatr Surg.*, 27(1), 83–90. doi: 10.4103/jiaps.JIAPS_334_20.
[117] Parmaksız, G., Noyan, A., Dursun, H., İnce, E., Anarat, R., and Cengiz, N. (2016). Role of new biomarkers for predicting renal scarring in vesicoureteral reflux: NGAL, KIM-1, and L-FABP. *Pediatr Nephrol.*, 31(1), 97–103. doi: 10.1007/s00467-015-3194-3.
[118] Nickavar, A., Valavi, E., Safaeian, B., and Moosavian, M. (2020). Validity of urine neutrophile gelatinase-associated lipocalin in children with primary vesicoureteral reflux. *Int Urol Nephrol.*, 52(4), 599–602. doi: 10.1007/s11255-019-02355-3.
[119] De Silva, P. M. C. S., Gunasekara, T. D. K. S. C., Gunarathna, S. D., Sandamini, P. M. M. A., Pinipa, R. A. I., Ekanayake, E. M. D. V., Thakshila, W. A. K. G., Jayasinghe, S. S., Chandana, E. P. S., and Jayasundara, N. (2021). Urinary biomarkers of renal injury KIM-1 and NGAL: Reference intervals for healthy pediatric population in Sri Lanka. *Children (Basel).*, 8(8), 684. doi: 10.3390/children8080684.
[120] Ning, M., Mao, X., Niu, Y., Tang, B., and Shen, H. (2018). Usefulness and limitations of neutrophil gelatinase-associated lipocalin in the assessment of kidney diseases. *J Lab Precis Med.*, 3, 1. doi: 10.21037/jlpm.2017.12.09.
[121] Biočić, M., Todorić, J., Budimir, D., Cvitković Roić, A., Pogorelić, Z., Jurić, I., and Šušnjar, T. (2012). Endoscopic treatment of vesicoureteral reflux in children with subureteral dextranomer/hyaluronic acid injection: A single-centre, 7-year experience. *Can J Surg.*, 55(5), 301–6. doi: 10.1503/cjs.003411.
[122] Läckgren, G., Cooper, C. S., Neveus, T., and Kirsch, A. J. (2021). Management of vesicoureteral reflux: What have we learned over the last 20 years? *Front Pediatr.*, 9, 650326. doi: 10.3389/fped.2021.650326.
[123] Ambarsari, C. G., Hidayati, E. L., Trihono, P. P., Saraswati, M., Rodjani, A., Wahyudi, I., Situmorang, G. R., Kim, J. J., Mellyana, O., and Kadaristiana, A. (2020). Experience of the first 6 years of pediatric kidney transplantation in Indonesia: A multicenter retrospective study. *Pediatr Transplant.*, 24(8), e13812. doi: 10.1111/petr.13812.
[124] Ambarsari, C. G., Cho, Y., Milanzi, E., Francis, A., Koh, L. J., Lalji, R., and Johnson, D. W. (2023). Epidemiology and outcomes of children with kidney failure receiving kidney replacement therapy in Australia and New Zealand. *Kidney Int Rep.*, 8(10), 1951–64. doi: 10.1016/j.ekir.2023.07.006.

Chapter 2

Standards for the Diagnostics and Treatment of Vesicoureteral Reflux in Children in the Russian Federation

Sergei Nikitin[1,2,*], **MD**
Natalia Guseva[3,4,5], **MD**
Svetlana Kononova[6]
and Vadim Nikitin[1]

[1]Medical institute, Petrozavodsk State University, Petrozavodsk, Russia
[2]Children's Republican Hospital named after I.N.Grigovich, Petrozavodsk, Russia
[3]Russian Medical Academy of Continuous Professional Education, Moscow, Russia
[4]Department of Pediatric Surgery Pirogov Medical University, Moscow, Russia
[5]Moscow Voiding Dysfunction Center Moscow Paediatric Speransky Hospital No. 9, Moscow, Russia
[6]Department of Pediatrics and Pediatric Surgery, Medical Institute of PetrSU, Petrozavodsk, Russia

Abstract

Vesicoureteral reflux is the most common type of uropathy in children, representing a considerable danger to patients due to possible complications, the most dangerous of which is pyelonephritis with an outcome in chronic renal failure. Considering the urgency of the problem and the plurality of opinions about the ways of its possible solution, the article describes the standards for the diagnostics and treatment of vesicoureteral reflux adopted in the Russian Federation. For the diagnostic of retrograde reflux of urine, various methods of examining the patient are used. It is possible to suspect the presence of reflux already

---

[*] Corresponding Author's Email: ssnikitin@yandex.ru.

In: Vesicoureteral Reflux
Editor: Garry M. Morones
ISBN: 979-8-89113-444-7
© 2024 Nova Science Publishers, Inc.

at the stage of collecting an anamnesis: the doctor should be alerted by complaints of urination disorders, recurrent urinary tract infections, episodes of fever to subfebrile values against the background of complete well-being; abdominal pain that cannot be associated with eating or defecation. In urine and blood tests, attention should be paid to changes that indicate the presence of inflammation. One of the markers of a possible reflux is an effective tool for diagnosing vesicoureteral reflux is the expansion of the pelvicalyceal system of the kidneys and ureter, which is detected by ultrasound of the urinary system. Carrying out ultrasonic pyelocystometry as an element of antenatal screening makes it possible to suspect vesicoureteral reflux at the stage of intrauterine development and plan the examination of the child at the postnatal stage. The most reliable way to diagnose vesicoureteral reflux is voiding cystography, this study also allows you to determine the degree of reflux, based on data on the severity of morphological changes in the upper urinary tract and the level of radiopaque reflux in them.

The main goal of treating vesicoureteral reflux is to prevent kidney complications. With the growth of the child, reflux often resolves on its own, in connection with this, the treatment of this pathology at low degrees of reflux is usually started with a regimen of corrective measures and antibiotic therapy for relapses of pyelonephritis. Methods of physiotherapeutic treatment are actively used: laser therapy, the use of paraffin and ozocerite on the bladder, sinusoidal modulating currents. Medical treatment of vesicoureteral reflux is most relevant when reflux is a complication of neurogenic bladder dysfunction, the most common form of which is an overactive bladder. If a conservative strategy fails, the next step in the treatment of vesicoureteral reflux is its surgical correction. The most common methods of surgical treatment are endoscopic intervention, which implies the introduction of a volume-forming substance under the mucous membrane of the ureter. With the ineffectiveness of several endoscopic corrections, laparoscopic, vesicoscopic, and open access operations are used. Of the open operations, the Cohen operation is most widely used. Currently, endoscopic correction is considered as an alternative to the appointment of permanent antibiotic therapy. Endoscopic treatment was previously performed only at low degrees of vesicoureteral reflux, Cohen's operation - at high, but now, to minimize surgical trauma, it is proposed to perform endoscopic correction in all patients as a measure of first-line surgical treatment.

Keywords: vesicoureteral reflux, reflux nephropathy, children

Introduction

Vesicoureteral (or vesicopelvic) reflux is the reflux of urine from the bladder into the ureters and into the pelvicalyceal system of the kidneys, due to a violation of the closing function of the ureterovesical fistula. The problem of vesicoureteral reflux is traditionally one of the most urgent in pediatric urology. The relevance of the issue is supported by the rather frequent dissatisfaction of practitioners with the possibilities of diagnosis and the results of treatment, the tendency to increase the degree of reflux with time and the development of complications: reflux nephropathy caused by backflow of urine into the kidney parenchyma; arterial hypertension and upper urinary tract infection [1-3]. Vesicoureteral reflux is the most common variant of uropathy in children, with girls being 4 times more common than boys. In this case, boys usually show a higher degree of reflux. It is also believed that in the population in 1% of children there is an "asymptomatic" vesicoureteral reflux that is not diagnosed and does not cause complications. But at the same time, in the etiology of chronic renal failure in children, reflux occupies 30-40% of cases [1, 3-4]. Given the relevance of the problem and the pluralism of opinions on how to solve it, in this article it was decided to highlight the standards for the diagnosis and treatment of vesicoureteral reflux that have been established in the Russian Federation.

Vesicoureteral reflux may be based on an anomaly in the development of the orifice of the ureter - its lateralization, neurogenic dysfunction of the bladder, and pronounced manifestations of cystitis. With lateralization of the orifice of the ureter, a shortening of the submucosal tunnel is revealed, the ratio of the diameter of the ureter to the length of the submucosal tunnel changes, the ratio of the length of the submucosal section of the ureter to the intramural one, as a result of which the closing function of the ureterovesical fistula becomes insufficient [4-5]. The cause of vesicoureteral reflux can also be other malformations of the urinary system: posterior urethral valve, bladder diverticulum, doubling and ureterocele [4].

The most common is vesicoureteral reflux, which develops as a result of neurogenic dysfunction of the bladder. Violation of the closing function of the ureterovesical fistula in this case is due to high intravesical pressure or atony of the bladder [3, 6]. High intravesical pressure develops with an overactive bladder, as well as with detrusor-sphincter dyssynergy [3]. It should be noted that the risk of developing vesicoureteral reflux and any complications from the upper urinary tract increases when intravesical pressure exceeds 40 cm H_2O. In this case, the normal passage of urine through the ureter is disturbed, intrapelvic pressure increases and glomerular filtration is disturbed [6]. With atony of the bladder, the closing function of the uretero-vesical anastomosis is disturbed due to a break in the peripheral nerves or pathways of the spinal cord. The bladder and ureters then represent a single reservoir with a constant flow of urine through the uretero-vesical fistula in both directions.

Vesicoureteral reflux can be both unilateral and bilateral, and the degree of reflux from different sides differs in about half of the cases. Depending on the frequency of reflux, it can be permanent or intermittent, the latter option significantly complicating the diagnosis of the disease [4, 6].

Gradation of vesicoureteral reflux is usually carried out depending on the severity of morphological changes in the upper urinary tract and the degree of reflux of the radiopaque substance in them, these indicators are evaluated during voiding cystography. The International Committee for the Study of Vesicoureteral Reflux adopted the Heikkel-Pozkulainen classification, which distinguishes five degrees of reflux [1, 6]:

- Grade 1 - reflux of the contrast agent only into the distal ureters without their expansion
- Grade 2 - the contrast agent reaches the renal calyces, while the urinary tract is not dilated
- Grade 3 - slight dilatation of the ureter and pyelocaliceal system
- Grade 4 - slight tortuosity of the ureter and a more significant expansion of the pelvis and calyces of the kidney, the contours of the calyces are smoothed
- Grade 5 - significant dilatation of the ureter and pyelocaliceal system, the ureter is tortuous, the contours of the renal calyces are smoothed.

With an increase in the degree of reflux, as a rule, the likelihood of complications also increases. However, sometimes nephrosclerosis develops regardless of the degree of reflux, which is associated with mutations in the TNFα (tumor necrosis factor, G308A mutation) and TGFβ (transforming growth factor) genes [4, 7].

It is possible to suspect vesicoureteral reflux already at the stage of collecting anamnesis. Clinically, the presence of vesicoureteral reflux can be suspected in case of urination disorders, with recurrent pain in the lumbar region and in the abdomen, which cannot be associated with eating or defecation; in the presence of a history of sudden rises in temperature to subfebrile values against the background of complete well-being; in the presence of signs of chronic intoxication, which is associated with a latent course of pyelonephritis in a child. Often, vesicoureteral reflux first manifests itself only with an attack of pyelonephritis or symptoms of serious secondary kidney damage - swelling and pallor of the skin, episodes of increased blood pressure (as an early symptom of reflux nephropathy occurs in more than 50% of cases [6]). When questioning a patient to assess the function of the lower urinary tract, it is important to pay attention to the frequency of urination, the need for tension in the abdominal muscles during micturition. In case of complaints of urinary incontinence, it is recommended to record a three-day urination diary (average effective volume and frequency of urination per day). Registration of a urination diary will suggest a possible variant of neurogenic bladder dysfunction [4, 8]. Often there are cases of combined dysfunction of the pelvic organs, the treatment of which should be complex, therefore, when collecting an anamnesis, it is mandatory to clarify the function of the rectum [5, 9]. A family history, burdened with diseases of the urinary system and, in particular, vesicoureteral reflux, can also help in making the correct diagnosis - according to Bataeva E.P. et al., the risk of inheriting vesicoureteral reflux reaches 30–50% [4].

On physical examination of the patient, there are no clinical signs of vesicoureteral reflux. But in patients with suspected vesicoureteral reflux, attention should be paid to the skin, mucous membranes - dryness, pallor can be detected, as signs of general intoxication in the latent course of pyelonephritis. Evaluate the presence of edema, the presence of which may indicate a decrease in kidney function. Palpation of the abdomen, lumbar region is performed to detect pain in the projection of the kidneys, ureters, and bladder. Examination of the external genital organs allows diagnosing associated anomalies. For vesicoureteral reflux, it is important to identify visible variants of infravesical obstruction: meatostenosis, meatus polyp, prolapse of the urethra, and sometimes prolapse of a part of the ureterocele [4].

Laboratory research methods can only indicate the presence of kidney damage and a decrease in their function, as well as the presence of inflammation of the urinary system. In a clinical blood test, a doctor should be alerted by an accelerated erythrocyte sedimentation rate and leukocytosis. The presence of anemia that is not amenable to standard treatment can be considered as a consequence of vesicoureteral reflux with the development of impaired renal function. In a biochemical blood test, a deviation from the norm in creatinine and urea indicates a decrease in kidney function, but these are late signs of the disease. A general urine test indicates the presence of inflammation in the urinary system. The functional state of the kidneys is also assessed using Reberg's tests with the calculation of glomerular filtration rate and Zimnitsky's test. To clarify the etiology of the inflammatory process with established vesicoureteral disease, it is recommended to carry out urine culture at least once every six months [4].

The most reliable way to diagnose vesicoureteral reflux is voiding cystography. During this study, a radiopaque substance is injected into the bladder through a catheter in the child's supine position. The introduction is carried out under the control of an electron-optical converter until the urge to urinate or until the age-related physiological capacity of the bladder is reached. Then two pictures are taken: the first - immediately after the injection of a contrast agent into the bladder, the second - during urination. Reflux can occur both in the phase of bladder emptying (active reflux) and in the phase of its filling (passive reflux) [1, 10]. In the first case, the tension of the detrusor during micturition causes an increase in intravesical pressure, which leads to the reflux of contrast agent into the ureters. This circumstance leaves vesicoureteral reflux a chance to go unnoticed if the child is unable to urinate during the study. In the second case, an increase in intravesical pressure and reflux can be caused, for example, by bladder overflow due to its hypoactivity [4].

The second way to diagnose vesicoureteral reflux is nephroscintigraphy with indirect cystography. Registration of

It is possible to suspect vesicoureteral reflux by indirect signs during an ultrasound examination. These signs are expansion of the pyelocaliceal system of the kidneys, thickening of the wall of the pelvis, expansion of the ureters, and detection of malformations with which reflux may be associated. For early diagnosis of reflux nephropathy, duplex scanning of renal blood flow is used [4].

Vesicoureteral reflux can be suspected already during an ultrasound examination at the stage of antenatal diagnosis. The most reliable anomalies of the kidneys are detected on the second screening ultrasound - at a gestational age of 22 weeks. Ultrasound examination reveals pyelectasis - an increase in the anterior-posterior diameter of the renal pelvis. In a study conducted by Deryugina L.A., to determine the presence of vesicoureteral reflux in the fetus, the method of ultrasonic dynamic pyelocystometry was used, the essence of which is to simultaneously determine the size of the renal pelvis and the volume of the bladder during one micturition cycle. The presence or absence of dependence of the size of the pelvis on the volume of the bladder spoke, respectively, of a functional or organic cause of obstruction of the upper urinary tract, which was a differential criterion for determining the cause of pyelectasis. The "stable pyelectasis" identified in this study during the postnatal examination of newborns was manifested by hydronephrosis caused by stenosis of the ureteral pelvis, or obstructive megaureter. In the group of children with "unstable" dilatation of the upper urinary tract during antenatal examination, vesicoureteral reflux was diagnosed during postnatal examination. In this case, the degree of reflux, defined in antenatal examination as intermittent visualization of the ureter, permanent visualization of the ureter, or permanent visualization with tortuosity, correlated with the degree of reflux in the neonatal period [3].

Another diagnostic criterion for vesicoureteral reflux is the visualization of ectopic and modified ureteral orifices and a reduced length of the intramural ureter during cystoscopy. So, in a study conducted by Solovyov A.E., a correlation was found between the degree of vesicoureteral reflux and the severity of morphological changes in the orifices of the ureters. The cystoscopic picture of grade 1 vesicoureteral reflux did not differ from that in the absence of pathologies: typical localization and shape of the orifices, the length of the submucosal ureter was more than 0.5 cm. With grade 2 vesicoureteral reflux, the localization and conformation of the orifices in most cases corresponded to normal, sometimes there were changes in the shape in the form of a horseshoe or arch. Vesicoureteral reflux of grades 3 and 4 was characterized by severe ectopia of the orifices and a change in their shape in the form of an arch or hole, the length of the intramural ureter is often less than 0.5 cm. The degree of vesicoureteral reflux was also compared with the severity of ectopia, for this, the zones of the location of the orifices of the ureters according to Lyon were used. Almost half of the children included in the study had a pronounced ectopia - the location of the orifices in zones B, C or D, outside the Lietaud triangle. In 9.8% of children, lateralization of the orifices was detected - location in zone A. In the remaining patients, localization was typical and corresponded to the norm - zones E and F. The work also established a correlation between the severity of ectopia of the orifices and the degree of renal hypoplasia [11].

Difficult in diagnostic terms is a variant of intermittent vesicoureteral reflux, which can often not be proven according to voiding cystography, but has characteristic signs in the form of recurrent urinary tract infections, ultrasound and radiological changes. In this case, the diagnosis is made on the basis of the above data after visualization of gaping ureteral orifices during cystoscopy [4].

If secondary vesicoureteral reflux is suspected in patients with dysfunctions of the lower urinary tract, urodynamic studies are performed: uroflowmetry, retrograde cystometry, urethral profilometry, and sometimes profilometry of the ureterovesical anastomosis. Of all the above, uroflowmetry is the most versatile and indispensable type of urodynamic study for diagnosing neurogenic dysfunctions of the lower urinary tract. When conducting uroflowmetry, such important indicators as the volume and time of urination are recorded. Based on these data, information is obtained about the flow rate and a uroflowmetric curve is recorded - the dependence of the volumetric flow rate (ml/s) on time. The normal shape of the curve is dome-shaped; in the presence of pathologies, a staccato-shaped curve, obstructive interrupted urination, rapid flow, a curve in the form of a plateau, etc. can be recorded. Different types of curves correspond to various disorders of the urodynamics of the lower urinary tract, which, together with their clinical manifestations, greatly simplifies the diagnostic search [4, 9]. Additional recording of the electrical activity of the pelvic floor muscles, simultaneous with uroflowmetry, can significantly expand its diagnostic capabilities - for example, this combination allows more accurate diagnosis of detrusor-sphincter dyssynergy [12].

Tactics of treatment of vesicoureteral reflux depends on its cause [5]. Currently, in Russia, various methods are used to treat retrograde reflux of urine: from regimen-corrective to surgical. In any case, the goal of reflux treatment is to preserve kidney function [1-2].

According to A. Yu. Pavlov et al., with the growth of the child, vesicoureteral reflux tends to self-resolve: in the case of reflux of the first or second degree, this occurs in 80% of cases, with the third degree - only in 40% of children. Age-related regression of reflux is associated with the physiological restructuring of the ureterovesical anastomosis: elongation of the intramural ureter, a change in the angle of its entry into the bladder, a decrease in diameter, and also with the stabilization of the bladder function [1, 5, 9]. According to Umalatova M.I., attributed to all causes of vesicoureteral reflux, by the age of 4-5 years, its spontaneous resolution is observed in 80% of cases for children with 2 degrees of reflux and in 30-50% for children with 3-4 degrees reflux [1].

When vesicoureteral reflux is detected against the background of neurogenic bladder dysfunction, treatment begins with behavioral therapy. It consists in the formation of adequate hydration and stimulation of the function of emptying the bladder. To do this, the child is offered to drink every 2 hours during wakefulness and empty the bladder after each fluid intake. Control the emptying of the rectum [13-14].

Drug treatment of vesicoureteral reflux is aimed at correcting the underlying disease, stabilizing the function of the bladder. The drugs of choice for the treatment of overactive bladder, as one of the most common forms of neurogenic dysfunctions of the lower urinary tract responsible for the development of reflux, are muscarinic cholinergic receptor blockers. The mechanism of action is based on the blockade of M-cholinergic receptors of the detrusor, which reduces its susceptibility to acetylcholine and levels out manifestations of overactivity - intravesical pressure decreases and bladder capacity increases. That is, there is a restoration of the cumulative function. The drugs of this group are used in oral form, but the option of their use by electrophoresis on the bladder area is also used. With detrusor-sphincter dyssynergy, drugs of the alpha-blocker group (doxazosin, tamsulosin) are used [9].

With a recurrent course of pyelonephritis, antibiotic therapy is prescribed. In the standard situation, 3rd generation cephalosporin antibiotics and nitrofurans are used. If a flora producing extended spectrum beta-lactamase is detected, the selection of an antibacterial drug is performed individually, according to the sensitivity of the microflora. Currently, extended-spectrum beta-lactamase producers stand out in 20% of positive urine cultures. The necessary duration of antibiotics is a debatable issue. With frequent and prolonged exacerbations of pyelonephritis, a scheme of prolonged antibiotic therapy for several months is justified [1].

Biofeedback therapy (BFB-therapy) is gaining popularity in Russia. When conducting biofeedback therapy, the equipment only registers the biological signals of the body, but does not have a direct effect on the child. To support motivation in children, during the procedure, they are shown an interactive video sequence on the screen, with which they can interact by regulating the activity of the pelvic floor muscles and the sphincter apparatus. The main task of biofeedback therapy is teaching self-regulation, physiological control of the muscles involved in the act of urination. The advantages of the method are non-invasiveness, treatment in a playful way, and ease of demonstrating the patient's success to the patient, which increases the motivation of children to continue the procedures [6, 13].

The effectiveness of biofeedback therapy was evaluated in a study that included 55 patients aged 4 to 17 years with dysfunctional urination or an overactive bladder, conducted by Morozov S. L. et al. Efficacy was assessed using the overactive bladder scale, the visual analogue scale, and the quality of life (QOL) scales. The QOL scale defines improvement in quality of life by the level of reduction in clinical symptoms: complete response - a decrease of more than 50%, partial response - a decrease of more than 25%, no response - a decrease of less than 25%. The effectiveness of the method in dysfunctional urination and overactive bladder was 79% and 78%, respectively, when assessing the dynamics of the disease 3 and 6 months after therapy, there was a significant improvement in the quality of life, a decrease in the level of residual urine [6].

Other methods of physiotherapeutic treatment of children with neurogenic bladder dysfunctions are also used. Their popularity is explained by the impact on all pathogenetic links of the disease and all levels of innervation of the bladder, the absence of side effects and the possibility of use in young children [15]. The method of dynamic electrical neurostimulation is widely used, the essence of which is the impact on the spinal centers of urination with pulsed currents, similar in shape and frequency to the action potentials of internal organs. The use of this technique in children with neurogenic dysfunctions of the bladder helps to increase the effective volume of the bladder and reduce intravesical pressure. The system of detrusor-stabilizing reflexes is affected by the method of anal stimulation with sinusoidal modulated and interference currents. Such currents have a low energy load and the possibility of a targeted impact on deeply located organs. Methods are used that improve the trophism of the detrusor, aimed at eliminating hypoxia and metabolic disorders in it. These methods include electro- and phonophoresis on the bladder area of drugs that improve microcirculation (eufillin, nicotinic acid). Heat therapy is considered an effective method of treating an overactive bladder. The positive effect is associated with thermal, chemical and mechanical effects on the area of the bladder ozokeritin, paraffin or mud applications [13]. To increase the effectiveness, methods of physiotherapy treatment are used in conjunction with physiotherapy exercises and massage, aimed at strengthening the muscles of the pelvic floor and the anterior abdominal wall. The type of vibromassage with the help of elastic pseudo-boiling layers is gaining popularity. The application of this method to the anorectal region contributes to the inhibition of bladder contractions through the system of detrusor-stabilizing reflexes [13].

Control examination is carried out in 6-12 months. When stopping detrusor overactivity, if vesicoureteral reflux persists, its endoscopic correction is performed [13, 14].

In Russia, both endoscopic methods of reflux treatment and open, laparoscopic and robotic types of surgical interventions are used [1-2].

Endoscopic method of treatment consists in the introduction of volume-forming substances under the mucous membrane of the intramural part of the ureter during cystoscopy [1-2]. This is necessary to create a dense base below the lumen of the ureter, which leads to an elongation of its intramural section. During micturition, intravesical pressure increases, and the upper wall of the ureter is pressed against the lower, lying on a dense basis - thus improving the closing function of the ureterovesical anastomosis [16]. Currently, 3 polymer injection techniques are used in Russia: STING (Subureteral Transurethral Injection), HIT1 (Hydrodistention Implantation Technique 1) and HIT2 (Hydrodistention Implantation Technique 2). The choice of technique is based on the degree of hydrodilation (H0-H3, H-hydrodilatation) of the orifices of the ureters, carried out during this study [17].

There are four degrees of hydrodilatation of the ureter [18]:

- H0 - the orifice of the ureter does not open when trying to hydrodilate
- H1 - the orifice of the ureter opens slightly during hydrodilatation, it is not possible to insert a cystoscope into the ureter
- H2 - the orifice of the ureter opens when trying to hydrodilate, it is possible to bring the cystoscope only into the intramural part of the ureter
- H3 - the orifice of the ureter opens when hydrodilatation is attempted, a full ureteroscopy is possible

According to 4 degrees of hydrodilation, 3 methods of introducing bulk-forming substances are used [17-18]:

1. STING - the introduction of the drug into the wall of the bladder directly under the orifice of the ureter
2. HIT1 - insufflation of the drug only directly into the wall of the distal part of the intramural ureter
3. HIT2 - injection of the drug into both the proximal and distal parts of the intramural ureter

Ureteral orifices with H0 and H1 degrees of hydrodilation can only be repaired using the traditional STING technique. When visualizing orifices with degrees of H2-H3 hydrodilation, it is possible to use all three described methods [17].

The issue of choosing the most effective volume-forming drug for endoscopic ureteroplasty is topical. The first ever drug used for endoscopic correction of reflux was Teflon paste. Despite the high efficiency of the use of this substance, a pronounced granulomatous reaction and the detection of polymer particles in the systemic circulation after administration forced researchers to embark on the path of finding another, safer drug. Currently, in Russia, the following substances are used for endoscopic ureteroplasty: collagen (of animal origin), DAM+ (consists of a three-dimensional polyacrylamide mesh polymer, purified water and silver ions), urodex (an analogue of the drug used in Russia and Europe "Deflux", consisting of microspheres of dextranomer and hyaluronic acid) and vantris (a preparation consisting of particles of a polyacrylate-polyalcohol copolymer immersed in a 40% glycerol solution). The drugs used do not cause a pronounced granulomatous reaction and do not migrate into the bloodstream [17, 19]. The effectiveness of these substances in the correction of vesicoureteral reflux was evaluated in a study conducted by Barseghyan E. R. et al., which included 831 children aged 4 months to 12 years. Children were divided into 4 groups depending on the drug used and the technique of its insufflation (STING, HIT1 and HIT2). The complete elimination of reflux was considered a positive result, and the effectiveness was evaluated after the first injection of a bulking agent. Group 1 included children who underwent collagen plasty according to the STING method - out of 216 treated ureters, a positive result was achieved only in 88 (40.7% of cases). Children of the second group underwent plastic surgery of the orifices with DAM+, a positive result was achieved in 68.7% of cases (212 ureters out of 309; using the STING technique, recovery was achieved in 60.7% of cases, HIT1 - 53.4%, HIT2 - 31.3%). In the third group of children, urodex was administered during endoscopic correction of reflux, a positive result was achieved in 69.5% of cases (with the use of the STING technique, recovery was achieved in 67.8% of cases, HIT1 - 61.4%, HIT2 - 58.6%). In group 4, plasty was performed with Vantris, a positive result was obtained in 78.5% of cases (using the STING method, recovery was achieved in 74.2% of cases, HIT1 - 69.8%, HIT2 - 62.3%.). Thus, urodex and vantris became the most effective drugs in reflux correction [17]. It is worth noting that some authors note the importance of the physical properties of polymers for the convenience of their introduction and the most accurate positioning, which provides reliable antireflux protection. Thus, preparations with a high density (vantris, teflon paste) are distributed locally, around the tip of the needle, while substances with a low density (DAM +, urodex) spread in the tissues without moving them apart, moreover, they are characterized by retrograde extrusion along needle during injection [19]. Taking into account the above features, Vantris is currently recognized as the most effective drug for endoscopic correction of vesicoureteral reflux [17, 19].

Another way to correct vesicoureteral reflux is to create a neoureterocystoanastomosis. The most common technique in Russia is the imposition of such an anastomosis according to Cohen. A vesicotomy is performed, the ureter is isolated, a submucosal tunnel is formed, into which the ureter is placed and a new mouth is formed. Ureterocystoanastomosis is accessible by vesicoscopic access: under cystoscopic control, three trocars are inserted into the bladder: the first port (6 mm) is installed through a puncture of the anterior abdominal wall approximately in the middle of the distance from the pubic symphysis to the navel, this port is used for optics; two other trocars are placed transrectally at the same distance to the right and left of the first port. The bladder is filled with carbon dioxide, the pressure is maintained at 12 mm. Hg. The ureter is excised with a sharp method, then a submucosal tunnel is formed in the bladder, and the ureter is passed into it. The bladder defect is sutured, and the distal end of the ureter is sutured to the bladder wall [2, 20].

The subject of active discussions is the choice of the method of surgical correction of vesicoureteral reflux. So, in a study conducted by Pirogov A. V. et al., the efficacy and safety of transurethral (endoscopic) and vesicoscopic surgery for primary retrograde reflux of urine in children were compared. A retrospective analysis of the results of treatment of 214 patients was carried out, divided into two groups: in the first group, all children underwent endoscopic correction of reflux, in the second - vesicoscopic ureterocystoanastomosis. Each group is divided into two subgroups: with low (grade 1–3) and high (grade 4–5) reflux. In most cases, the indications for surgery were recurrent urinary tract infections; in some cases, the reason for surgery was progressive reflux nephropathy. The study included both unilateral and bilateral variants of vesicoureteral reflux. It should be noted that the age of children in the group of endoscopic correction was significantly lower than the age of children in the group of vesicoscopic interventions (53.5 ± 44.4 months versus 72.0 ± 50.4 months). Urinary tract infections and bilateral reflux were also more common in the endoscopic treatment group [2].

In the group of children who underwent endoscopic intervention, in the subgroup with grades 1-3 refluxes, after the first injection of polyacrylate copolymer, complete elimination of retrograde urinary reflux was achieved in 91.7% of cases. One patient required a second injection of a volume-forming drug to completely eliminate reflux. After the treatment, contralateral reflux developed in 12.8% of children. In the group of patients with reflux of the same degree and the Cohen operation performed, reflux was eliminated in 100% of cases, the formation of contralateral reflux was not observed in any of the patients. Postoperative complications for patients of the first group were obstruction of the urtero-vesical segment and recurrence of vesicoureteral reflux. In children of the second group, complications were obstruction of the ureterovesical segment, migration of the external drainage of the ureter into the bladder, foreign bodies of the bladder, and the development of perivesical hematoma. In patients with grade 4–5 reflux and endoscopic intervention after the first injection of a volume-forming substance, reflux stopped in 76.3% of cases. After the second administration of the drug to a number of patients, this number increased to 81.4%. Contralateral vesicoureteral reflux developed in 13.3% of cases. In patients with a high degree of reflux and ureterocystoanastomosis, complete elimination of urine reflux into the upper urinary tract was achieved in 100% of cases, contralateral reflux was formed in 6.9% of patients. Among the patients of the first group, postoperative complications were obstruction of the ureterovesical segment and recurrence of vesicoureteral reflux. In the second group, patients developed acute obstruction of the ureterovesical segment, in one case the complication was urine leakage from the trocar access [2].

Thus, Cohen's operation has always proved to be more effective than endoscopic administration of a volume-forming agent. However, taking into account the invasiveness of vesicoscopic surgery, as well as its longer duration compared to endoscopic intervention (average 100 minutes versus 15) and the need for longer hospitalization (average 5 days versus 2), the authors concluded that at low degrees of reflux (grade 1-3), endoscopic correction is preferred. The choice of tactics of surgical treatment, in their opinion, should be based on the division of refluxes into high and low degrees [2].

On the other hand, taking into account the lower than with low-grade reflux, but still high efficiency of endoscopic treatment of vesicoureteral reflux at grades 4–5, some authors quite reasonably suggest this method of correction as a measure of first-line surgical treatment for all refluxes. The transition to an extensive surgical technique involving reimplantation of the ureter is possible, in their opinion, only after the second unsuccessful attempt at endoscopic treatment. So, in a study conducted by S. N. Zorkin et al., a positive result of endoscopic correction of grade 4–5 reflux (complete elimination of reflux or reduction to grade 1) after the first injection of a volume-forming drug was achieved in 68.7% of cases. Among the remaining patients after the second attempt to bring volume-forming substances under the mouth of the ureters, a positive result was achieved in 48.9% of children.

Patients for whom endoscopic treatment proved to be ineffective were operated on according to the Cohen or Politano-Leatbetter methods. Thus, endoscopic intervention in all patients with vesicoureteral reflux as the first line of surgical treatment avoids unnecessary trauma to patients [10].

Operation by the Lich-Gregoir technique is possible with laparoscopic access, and this operation is also used in rare cases of ineffectiveness of the Cohen operation. Its peculiarity lies in extravesical access - a submucosal tunnel is created by dissecting the bladder muscle from the outside.

Conclusion

Vesicoureteral reflux is a common condition in the pediatric population. Its danger lies in the formation of pyelonephritis, dilatation of the kidney collectors, which ultimately leads to the development of chronic renal failure. It is possible to suspect the presence of vesicoureteral reflux already during an ultrasound examination of pregnant women. In this case, after birth, a urological examination of the child is performed, obstructive uropathy is excluded. In a newborn child, it is fundamentally important to identify and eliminate the most serious malformations - the valve of the posterior urethra, a large ureterocele. Upon restoration of urodynamics in such cases, within a few months, vesicoureteral reflux is prone to spontaneous resolution. In the neonatal period, it is not recommended to perform operations for vesicoureteral reflux. In the first 2-3 weeks of a child's life, a very differentiated approach should be taken to the appointment of X-ray contrast studies due to the possible nephrotoxicity of drugs containing iodine.

Subsequently, vesicoureteral reflux can be detected when examining children with urination disorders, with leukocyturia, or when pyelectasis is detected on ultrasound. Conservative treatment of vesicoureteral reflux is most effective in neurogenic bladder and cystitis - its spontaneous resolution occurs in the treatment of the underlying disease. With lateralization of the orifice of the ureter, the most effective surgical treatment is endoscopic correction or neoimplantation of the ureter. In case of recurrent course of pyelonephritis against the background of vesicoureteral reflux, endoscopic correction is applied. It reduces the frequency of recurrence of pyelonephritis and the duration of antibiotic therapy.

This study was performed using the Unique Scientific Unit (UNU) «Multicomponent software and hardware system for automated collection, storage, markup of research and clinical biomedical data, their unification and analysis based on Data Center with Artificial Intelligence technologies» (reg. number: 2075518)

References

[1] Umalatova, M. I., Lefitov, G. M., and Maxachev, B. M. (2018). «Vesicoureteral reflux in children: clinic, diagnosis and approaches to therapy». *Sovremennaya nauka: aktual`ny`e problemy` teorii i praktiki* [*Modern science: current problems of theory and practice*], 6, 230-233. (in Russ.)

[2] Pirogov, A. V., Sizonov, V. V., and Kogan, M. I. (2020). «Comparative efficacy and safety of transurethral and vesicoscopic surgery for primary vesicoureteral reflux in children». *Vestnik urologii* [*Herald of urology*], 8, 58–68. (in Russ.)

[3] Deryugina, L. A. (2018). «Vesicoureteral reflux and its prenatal prognosis». Pediatriya im. G.N. Speranskogo [Pediatrics named after G.N. Speransky], 97 (5), 14–19. DOI: 10.24110/0031-403X2018-97-5-14-19. (in Russ.)

[4] Bataeva, E. P., and Zeleneva, A. Yu. (2019). «Vesicoureteral reflux in children - diagnostic issues». *Zabajkal`skij medicinskij zhurnal* [*Transbaikal Medical Journal*], 3, 9–12. (in Russ.)

[5] Pavlov, A. Yu., Maslov, S. A., Polyakov, N. V., Lisenok, A. A., and Simonyan, G. V. (2006). «*Vesicoureteral reflux in children: treatment tactics*», 7, 16. (in Russ.)

[6] Morozov, S. L., Dlin, V. V., and Shabel`nikova, E. I. (2020). «Biofeedback method in children with dysfunctional urination and overactive bladder, complicated by urinary incontinence, vesicoureteral reflux, nephropathy». *Praktika pediatra* [*Practice of a pediatrician*], 2, 33–40. (in Russ.)

[7] Shaxnovskij, D. S., Zorkin, S. N., Savost`yanov, K. V., Pushkov, A. A., and Burdenny`j, A. M. (2018). «Study of the association of TNFa, INFy, and TGFp gene polymorphisms with the risk of developing vesicoureteral reflux in children in the Russian population». *Pediatriya named after GN Speransky*, 97 (5), 79-84. DOI: 10.24110/0031-403X-2018-97-5-79-84. (in Russ.)

[8] Omurbekov, T. O., Arbanaliev, M. K., Poroshhaj, V. N., E`miroslanova, S. S., and Xegaj, E. V. (2022). «Treatment of various forms of neurogenic bladder dysfunction in children». *Vestnik KGMA imeni I. K. Axunbaeva* [*Newspaper KGMA named after I. K. Aknbaeva*], 4 (4), 93–100. DOI: 10.54890/1694-6405_2022_4_93. (in Russ.)

[9] Vorob`eva, Yu. D., Sy`t`kov, V. V., Zokirov, N. Z., Bushueva, T. V., Yacyk, S. P., and Fedorova, E. V. (2020). «Overactive bladder in children: new in diagnosis and treatment». *Rossijskij pediatricheskij zhurnal* [*Russian pediatric magazine*], 23(5), 330-334. DOI: 10.18821/1560-9561-2020-23-5-330-334. (in Russ.)

[10] Zorkin, S. N., Shaxnovskij, D. S., Turov, F. O., Galuzinskaya, A. T., and D`yakonova, E. Yu. (2020). «The effectiveness of endoscopic correction of high-grade vesicoureteral reflux in children». *Detskaya xirurgiya* [*Children's surgery*], 24 (5), 292-296. DOI: 10.18821/1560-9510-2020-24-5-292-296. (in Russ.)

[11] Solov`ev, A. E. (2022). «Cystoscopy in the diagnosis of vesicoureteral reflux of hyperplastic kidneys in children». Vyatskij medicinskij vestnik [*Vyatka medical journal*], 1(73), 19-23. DOI: 10.24412/2220-7880-2022-1-19-23. (in Russ.)

[12] Guseva, N. B., Nikitin, S. S., Ignat`ev, R. O., and Bozhendaev, T. L. (2019). «Incomplete bladder emptying syndrome in children: spectrum of differential diagnosis». *Pediatriya named after GN Speransky* [*Pediatrics named after GN Speranskyi*], 98 (5), 8-14. (in Russ.)

[13] Novikova, E. V. (2018). «Treatment and medical rehabilitation of children with overactive bladder». Rossijskij vestnik detskoj xirurgii, anesteziologii i reanimatologii [*Russian Bulletin of Pediatric Surgery, Anesthesiology and Reanimatology*], 8 (4), 105-110. DOI: 10.30946/2219-4061-2018-8-4-105-110. (in Russ.)

[14] Guseva, N. B., Nikitin, S. S., Varlamova, T. V., and Zaripova, Yu. R. (2020). Vesicoureteral reflux in combination with dysfunction of the pelvic organs in an 8-year-old child. *Pediatriya named after GN Speransky*, 96 (5), (in Russ.)

[15] Novikova, E. V., Xan, M. A., and Menovshhikova, L. B. (2020). «The use of laser radiation and interference currents in the medical rehabilitation of children with neurogenic bladder dysfunction». Voprosy` kurortologii, fizioterapii i lechebnoj fizicheskoj kul`tury` [Questions about balneology, physiotherapy and physical therapy], 98 (4), 71-76. DOI: 10.38025/ 2078–1962– 2020–98–4–71–76. (in Russ.)

[16] Burkin, A. G., Yacyk, S. P., Sharkov, S. M., Rusakov, A. A., and Tin, I. F. (2014). «Endoscopic treatment of vesicoureteral reflux in children». *Urologiya*, 5, 102-106. (in Russ.)

[17] Barsegyan, E. R., and Zorkin, S. N. (2014). «Comparative evaluation of the effectiveness of the use of various polymers in endoscopic correction of vesicoureteral reflux in children». *Detskaya xirurgiya* [*Children's surgery*], 18 (5), 4-8. (in Russ.)

[18] Cerwinka, W. H., Scherz, H. C., and Kirsch, A. J. (2008). Dynamic hydrodistention classification of the ureter and the double hit method to correct vesicoureteral reflux. *Archivos Espanoles de Urologia* [*Spanish Archives of Urology*], 61 (8), 882-887.

[19] Abdullaev, F. K., Kulaev, V. D., and Nikolaev V. V. (2013). «Dependence of the effectiveness of endoscopic treatment of primary vesicoureteral reflux on volume-forming material». *Urologiya*, 2, 94-97. (in Russ.)

[20] Pirogov, A. V., Sizonov, V. V., and Kogan, M. I. (2017). «Experience of 157 vesicoscopic operations in children». *Urologiya*, 6, 59-64. (in Russ.)

Chapter 3

When Does Vesicoureteral Reflux Develop in Children Operated on for a Spinal Hernia?

Sergei Nikitin[1,2,*], MD
Natalia Guseva[3,4,5,†], MD
Svetlana Kononova[6]
and Vadim Nikitin[1,‡]

[1]Medical institute, Petrozavodsk State University, Petrozavodsk, Russia
[2]Children's Republican Hospital named after I. N. Grigovich, Petrozavodsk, Russia
[3]Russian Medical Academy of Continuous Professional Education, Moscow, Russia
[4]Department of Pediatric Surgery Pirogov Medical University, Moscow, Russia
[5]Moscow Voiding Dysfunction Center Moscow Paediatric Speransky Hospital No. 9, Moscow, Russia
[6]Department of Pediatrics and Pediatric Surgery, Medical Institute of PetrSU, Petrozavodsk, Russia

Abstract

Spinal hernias occur with a frequency of 1-2:1000 newborns, more often localized in the lumbosacral region. Spinal hernias are often found in the structure of combined malformations and can also be combined with more than 40 chromosomal abnormalities. Spinal neurogenic bladder is the most severe consequence of spinal hernias. Spinal voiding dysfunctions develop due to underdevelopment of the terminal part of the spinal cord. In addition, prolonged compression of the spinal cord and cauda eqina during intrauterine development is of great importance. And

---

[*] Corresponding Author's Email: ssnikitin@yandex.ru.
[†] Corresponding Author's Email: guseva-n-b@yandex.ru.
[‡] Corresponding Author's Email: vadimnikitin11@yandex.ru.

In: Vesicoureteral Reflux
Editor: Garry M. Morones
ISBN: 979-8-89113-444-7
© 2024 Nova Science Publishers, Inc.

a significant contribution to the development of dysfunction is also made by intraoperative destruction of nerve structures during the correction of a spinal hernia. In almost all patients, in addition to voiding dysfunction, there is also a violation of emptying of the rectum due to innervation of the pelvic organs from the same sources and a single blood supply. Violations of pelvic functions, as a rule, appear at birth or immediately after surgery and in the future require lifelong support of a urologist. At the same time, there is currently no treatment method that could ensure a full recovery.

In addition to the manifestations of the neurogenic bladder itself, urologists face its complications in many patients. In terms of prevalence, infection of the urinary system comes out on top. In our patients, infection of the urinary system with spinal neurogenic bladder occurred in 98% of cases and manifested itself in the form of pyelonephritis, cystitis or a combination of them. The recurrence of pyelonephritis is associated with the formation of nephrosclerosis and the development of chronic renal failure. In this regard, it is necessary to carefully monitor the biochemical parameters in patients with spinal neurogenic bladder – to monitor the levels of urea, creatinine, microalbuminuria.

The second most common complication of spinal neurogenic bladder is vesicoureteral reflux. Certain urodynamic conditions are necessary for the formation of vesicourethonic reflux in spinal neurogenic bladder. First of all, this is high intravesical pressure, which can manifest itself in the form of high basic intravesical pressure or in the form of non-inhibited detrusor contractions against the background of normal base pressure. The second is a spasm of the urethral sphincter (and pelvic floor muscles). In this case, to ensure the act of urination, the detrusor is forced to develop an even higher intravesical pressure, and intra-abdominal pressure is also connected. Against the background of such variants of detrusor hypertension, the closing function of the uretero-vesical anastomosis is disrupted, and vesicoureteral reflux is formed.

There are variants of spinal neurogenic bladder, in which vesicoureteral reflux practically does not occur - this is the atony of the detrusor and sphincter. In such a situation, all the urine that enters the bladder immediately flows out through the urethra. With detrusor atony and hyperactivity of the sphincter, high-grade vesicoureteral reflux is often detected – with enlargement of the ureter, kidney pelvis and calyx. In this situation, the entire system of kidney collectors together with the bladder is a single reservoir and first of all it is necessary to solve the issue of adequate urine drainage.

The article presents treatment regimens for spinal neurogenic bladder and its complications – vesicoureteral reflux. Catheterization schemes depending on the variant of neurogenic bladder are presented. Intermittent and permanent catheterization of the bladder, conditions for reducing the frequency of catheterization and rejection of it are described. In addition, treatment regimens with M-holinoblockers for neurogenic detrusor hyperactivity are presented. Among the M-cholinoblockers, trospium chloride, oxybutynin hydrochloride, tolterodine and other means are currently used. In addition to M-cholinoblockers, alpha-blockers are used in the treatment of spinal neurogenic bladder. Metabolic drugs are also used. The methods of physiotherapy are described – with detrusor hyperactivity relaxing techniques on the bladder, and with atony – stimulating.

Keywords: children, spinal neurogenic bladder, neurogenic detrusor overactivity, atonic bladder, underactive bladder, urodynamics, vesicoureteral reflux

Operations for spinal hernias have long been part of the routine practice of neurosurgeons. The quality of these interventions and outcomes are constantly improving. The most severe consequence of a spinal hernia is a spinal neurogenic bladder. It is this condition that leads to the disability of patients and to date there is no treatment method that could ensure a full recovery. Spinal voiding dysfunctions develop due to underdevelopment of the terminal part of the spinal cord. In addition, prolonged compression of the spinal cord and cauda eqina during intrauterine development is of great importance. And a significant contribution to the development of dysfunction is made by intraoperative destruction of nerve structures during the correction of a spinal hernia. In almost all patients, in addition to voiding dysfunction, there is also a violation of emptying of the rectum due to innervation of the pelvic organs from the same sources and a single blood supply. Violations of pelvic functions, as a rule, appear at birth or immediately after surgery and in the future require lifelong support of a urologist.

Spinal hernias develop at the gestation period of 3-4 weeks. In the Russian Federation, all pregnant women undergo ultrasound examination of the fetus at 10-14, 20-22 and 34 weeks of gestation. The purpose of early prenatal diagnosis is to identify fetal malformations. Early detection of spinal hernias is a difficult task. The minimum possible period of ultrasound diagnosis of this anomaly is considered to be 9-10 weeks [1], and the reliable period is 14-16 weeks of gestation – when visualizing the ossification points of the posterior vertebrae. Ultrasound examination is a method of primary diagnosis and in cases where its capabilities do not allow unambiguously identifying the detected changes, an additional method of investigation is magnetic resonance imaging [2]. It is possible to detect a spinal hernia by magnetic resonance imaging in the second and third trimester of pregnancy in 100% of cases [3].

Spinal hernias occur with a frequency of 1-2:1000 newborns, more often localized in the lumbosacral region. Spinal hernias are often found in the structure of combined malformations and can also be combined with more than 40 chromosomal abnormalities [4]. If a spinal hernia is detected during ultrasound examination, future parents are explained about all the consequences of this malformation, especially about the inevitability of urological disorders, paresis and paralysis of the legs. The decision to prolong or terminate pregnancy is made, of course, by the parents, and if the parents decide to prolong pregnancy, the fetal urodynamics is assessed by monitoring the process of filling and emptying the bladder during ultrasound examination [5]. With myelodysplasia, a violation of the function of the bladder occurs in utero, so it is necessary to determine the condition of the upper urinary tract as early as possible, their possible damage. Ultrasound examination of the kidneys is performed in the first 5-7 days after delivery. Examination of the urinary system of a child with a spinal hernia after birth is aimed at detailing the presence of independent urination, residual urine, detection of megaureter, ectasia of the pelvis of the kidneys, assessment of the state of the parenchyma, its blood supply. It is necessary to clarify the state of the bladder, its dysfunction manifests itself in the form of an unhardened bladder, detrusor-sphincter dissinergia and / or urinary incontinence with pelvic floor paralysis and sphincter apparatus. The main pathological conditions leading to damage to the upper urinary tract in children with myelodysplasia are high intravesical pressure, muscle contraction of the urethral sphincter during urination and chronic urinary retention. In conditions of such pathological urodynamics, vesicoureteral reflux (up to 50% of patients), repeated exacerbations of chronic pyelonephritis and functional obstruction of urine outflow into the bladder appear, which leads to the development of chronic renal failure [4].

If a spinal hernia is operated on in the first few days after birth, then before the operation, urine is removed by means of a permanent catheter. After catheter extraction, urodynamics is examined in the postoperative period. The possibility and frequency of urination are determined - the presence of a stream of urine or its constant release by drops, effective and residual volumes, the presence of difficulty urinating (with anxiety, straining, intermittent nature of urine flow). In addition, the presence of constipation and encopresis is detected. The level of spinal lesion does not always correspond to clinical data in children.

Performing cystometry, urethral profilometry is possible at any age, but the most adequate urodynamic study can be performed at an age when a child can cooperate with a researcher during the procedure – indicate the presence of an urge, perform a cough test, perform uroflowmetry. We believe that such an opportunity appears after 3 years. Up to this age, measurement of intravesical and urethral pressure, measurement of bladder capacity are available. With spinal neurogenic bladder, the sensitivity of the perineum is more often reduced, which to a certain extent facilitates the procedure of urodynamic examination. The study of urodynamics makes it possible to clarify the state of the detrusor and sphincter. Understanding the features of urodynamics in a patient with a neurogenic bladder allows you to choose the best option for urine drainage. The choice of the method of urine removal should contribute to maintaining remission of urinary tract infection and prevent or delay the appearance of chronic renal failure. The simplest, most affordable and least risky method of urine removal is intermittent catheterization of the bladder, which allows the evacuation of residual urine. Effective emptying of the bladder promotes adequate emptying of the ureters and pelvis of the kidneys during their ectasia, preventing their infection and, in the future, the occurrence of recurrent infections of the urinary system. It should be noted that even with optimal treatment and the implementation of all recommendations, complications in the form of infection of the urinary system are almost inevitable. In our patients, infection of the urinary system with spinal neurogenic bladder occurred in 98% of cases and manifested itself in the form of pyelonephritis, cystitis or a combination of them.

According to the international classification recommended by the European Society of Urology (2010), there are:

- overactive blader with high intravesical pressure, reduced capacity and elasticity;
- underactive blader with low intravesical pressure, weakening or lack of effective contractions.

The sphincter apparatus (internal and external sphincters) can be:

- overactive, causing functional obstruction (detrusor-sphincter dyssinergia);
- be in a state of paralysis, without creating resistance to the flow of urine.

These states can be combined in various ways [4].

E. L. Vishnevsky [6] in the description of urodynamic disorders in neurogenic bladder identified two syndromes. The first is a small (spastic) bladder, characterized by a violation of the somatic innervation of the external urethral, anal sphincters and pelvic floor muscles; a decrease in the reservoir function of the bladder; mainly combined urinary incontinence; intravesical hypertension; a minimal number of complications from the upper urinary tract.

The second is the syndrome of incomplete emptying of the bladder: the reservoir function is not impaired, changes in the parasympathetic innervation of the bladder and the emptying phase are detected; the urge to urinate is reduced or absent, emptying of the bladder is incomplete, a large amount of residual urine; incontinence - by the type of paradoxical ischuria; in 2/3 of patients, severe lesions of the upper urinary tract are detected.

N. Madersbacher [7] presented a scheme of lesion levels in the nervous system depending on the urodynamic variant of the neurogenic bladder, in which the state of detrusor and sphincter is determined (overactive, normoactive and underactive, their various combinations).

Depending on the type of dysfunction, therapy is used to optimize the function of filling and emptying the bladder. The gold standard in the treatment of detrusor overactivity are drugs of the M-cholinoblokers group. Anticholinergic drugs help to reduce vesical pressure and increase the capacity of the bladder. With a underactive bladder, the main direction is to stimulate detrusor tone, anticholinesterase agents are used. The presence of incomplete emptying of the bladder determines the need for intermittent catheterization of the bladder. In parallel with the mediator drugs, the means of metabolic therapy are prescribed. Officially, the means of metabolic therapy for neurogenic bladder are off-label drugs. It is difficult to prove the effectiveness of these drugs in a scientific discussion. However, as activators of energy metabolism, these funds are widely used by neurologists in the Russian Federation.

High risks of impaired renal function determine the need for constant monitoring of its function. Quantitative determination of creatinine, serum urea, glomerular filtration rate, presence of microalbuminuria and metabolic acidosis is used to assess the condition of the glomeruli and tubules of the kidneys. Microalbuminuria is a marker of the risk of chronic kidney disease. The glomerular filtration rate and microalbuminuria determine the function of the glomeruli, and metabolic acidosis is a marker of damage to the tubules, and can also be detected in obstructive uropathies. Metabolic acidosis appears already with renal insufficiency. Microalbuminuria and metabolic acidosis are more often detected in dynamics, against the background and despite adequate therapy [8].

Below we will focus on the main problems of the patient, which are usually voiced by parents when they first contact a neurologist. The main problem is the violation of the act of urination. They manifest themselves in the form of:

- constant flow of urine in drops and / or in the form of a small jet of 5-15 ml every few minutes, while at least some formed act of urination is absent;
- in addition, there may be the presence of chronic urinary retention, which determines the need to catheterize the bladder every 3-4 hours from an early age – when the equivalent of an urge appears, most often in the form of abdominal pain;
- sometimes there is an act of urination – 20-80 ml of urine is released, but after 10-90 minutes after urination, urine begins to leak in drops.

The second most common problem of patients is recurrent infection of the urinary system, which can manifest itself both in the form of frequent exacerbations of pyelonephritis with intoxication, fever, and subclinically – only in the form of leukocyturia.

The third most frequent manifestation is constipation, encopresis, which parents correct with the help of various mechanical aids – pressing on the stomach, on the perineum on the sides of the anus to facilitate the evacuation of the contents of the rectum, with the help of enemas, mechanical cleansing of the rectal ampoule with a finger.

Usually, before contacting a neurologist, children are already being examined in urological, nephrological or pediatric departments of hospitals, where the main diagnostic complex is carried out, including ultrasound, microvision cystography and intravenous urography, as well as urine tests. At the same time, the main urological methods in almost half of patients reveal vesicoureteral reflux, pyelectasia, less often - megaureter. Correction of vesicoureteral reflux in spinal neurogenic bladder both operatively and conservatively is extremely difficult and ineffective until the detrusor function is stabilized.

Before starting the selection of treatment for children with spinal neurogenic bladder, it is mandatory to conduct a neurological - urodynamic study. Diagnosis of the functional state of the detrusor is possible by cystometry, and the sphincter by urethral profilometry. A complementary method is uroflowmetry, but its implementation is most often impossible due to the absence of an arbitrary act of urination. According to the results of the urodynamic study in children with spinal neurogenic bladder, it is advisable to distinguish two main groups – patients with atonic areflective bladder and children with neurogenic detrusor overactivity – these are opposite detrusor states that will require completely different therapeutic tactics. Each group is divided according to the condition of the external urethral sphincter: overactive or insufficiency. Neurogenic detrusor overactivity, depending on its manifestations, can be divided into two subgroups – patients with high baseline intravesical pressure and with non-inhibited contractions of the bladder against the background of normal baseline pressure.

In this article, we want to consider options for spinal voiding dysfunctions, in which vesicoureteral reflux develops. The main urodynamic conditions for the development of vesicoureteral reflux are high intravesical pressure and functional infravesical obstruction - spasm of the pelvic floor muscles. At the same time, the greatest risks of developing vesicoureteral reflux occur with the simultaneous manifestation of these two factors.

Let's analyze the variants of dysfunction with neurogenic detrusor overactivity. The latter can manifest itself in the form of high baseline intravesical pressure and in the presence of non-inhibited detrusor contractions against the background of normal baseline intravesical pressure. In each group there are differences in the state of the sphincter – overactive or insufficiency. Variants of neurogenic detrusor overactivity are important in terms of the intensity of therapy, predicting the effectiveness of treatment, although the therapy itself is identical. The experience of treating this category of patients has shown that in the presence of high baseline intravesical pressure, it is more difficult to correct hypertension. In this situation, almost constant intake of M-cholinoblockers is required and the dose of drugs used will be higher than with normal basic intravesical pressure with non-inhibited detrusor contractions. Among M-cholinoblockers, trospium chloride, oxybutynin hydrochloride, tolterodine and others are used. The dosage of M-cholinoblockers is selected individually, the general is the need for courses of therapy with short breaks in treatment. In the presence of high basic intravesical pressure, a course is usually prescribed for 3 weeks, then a break of 3-5 days, then a repeat course, and so on. The treatment regimen also includes an alpha-adrenoblocker (for 7 out of 12 months with interruptions). This tactic allows you to reduce the base pressure to standard values (below 20 cm H_2O). With a longer than 5 days break in taking the M-cholinoblocker, the base intravesical pressure begins to rise again.

In the presence of non-inhibited detrusor contractions, breaks in taking M–cholinoblockers are longer, the following scheme is possible: 6 weeks of admission - 1 month break. With a decrease in the number and pressure of non-inhibited contractions, breaks in taking the drug can increase up to 6 weeks. The alpha-adrenoblocker can be used according to the following scheme: 2 months reception, then 1.5-2 months break.

With both variants of neurogenic detrusor overactivity, it is possible to perform chemodenervation of the bladder by introducing botulinum toxin into the detrusor to reduce the dosages and frequency of use of M-cholinoblockers. Of the general methods of treatment for patients with neurogenic detrusor overactivity, regardless of the state of the sphincter, paraffin and a magnetolaser for the bladder, a preparation of magnesium and pyridoxine hydrochloride, L-carnitine, coenzyme Q10 are used.

There is a fundamental difference in treatment depending on the state of the sphincter. The state of the sphincter in neurogenic detrusor overactivity differentiates treatment tactics. Neurogenic detrusor overactivity with overactive state of the sphincter is the condition most in need of catheterization of the bladder due to the pronounced load on the kidneys – due to the detection of vesicoureteral reflux in more than half of patients and the recurrent course of pyelonephritis. Intermittent catheterization of the bladder is started, usually every 3 hours. Only against the background of a persistent decrease in intravesical pressure, it is possible to reduce the frequency of catheterizations of the bladder. An indicator of the effectiveness of treatment is the improvement of urine flow (the appearance of functionally obstructive urination, obstructive intermittent urination - with less use of abdominal muscles) and more effective emptying of the bladder with the amount of residual urine not exceeding 15%, relief of vesicoureteral reflux and remission of pyelonephritis. Physiotherapy used in the treatment of overactivity of the sphincter consists in conducting courses of paraffin therapy, biofeedback therapy, acupuncture.

Patients with neurogenic detrusor overactivity and insufficiency of the urethral sphincter experience less need for intermittent catheterization of the bladder. But this particular group of patients is more in need of finding the "golden mean" between the dose of the M-cholinoblocker, the frequency of catheterizations of the bladder and the alpha-adrenoblocker regimen. With an increase in the dose of the M-cholinoblocker, against the background of a decrease in intravesical pressure and continued stimulation of the pelvic floor, urine leakage stops, but the residual volume of the bladder increases, requiring increased catheterization. In this group of patients, the minimum possible dose of the M-cholinoblocker is selected to maintain low intravesical pressure, which makes it possible to form an act of urination.

Treatment of a child with neurogenic spinal bladder complicated by vesicoureteral reflux is carried out constantly and daily. With the correct and complete implementation of all medical recommendations, it is possible to stop vesicoureteral reflux with conservative measures. According to our data, 75% of cases manage to do without surgical treatment. In 25% of children with persistent vesicoureteral reflux, we perform endoscopic correction.

Despite the entire arsenal of medical, behavioral, physiotherapy and bladder catheterization used, children may be resistant to treatment and even the urodynamic situation may worsen. At the same time, it is necessary to think about the possible fixation of the spinal cord by the scar-adhesive process in the spinal canal, which requires repeated surgical treatment. In this situation, monitoring of magnetic resonance imaging of the lumbosacral region is necessary. If the fixed spinal cord is confirmed, then it is advisable to postpone measures aimed at restoring the function of the bladder until surgical treatment on the spinal canal, using only intermittent, and in some cases, permanent catheterization of the bladder.

A different situation develops with bladder atony – an extreme variant of detrusor underactivity. The intravesical pressure in such a bladder always remains low. The condition of the bladder itself in this situation does not create prerequisites for the development of vesicoureteral reflux. The state of the urethral sphincter matters. With his overactivity, we are faced with a situation that is designated as ishuria paradoxa – incontinence by drops with chronic urinary retention. With this variant of neurogenic bladder, we observed vesicoureteral reflux in 32% of patients. We believe that reflux here is associated with dilation and atony of the ureterovesical anastomosis. The degree of vesicoureteral reflux in this variant of neurogenic bladder, as a rule, is high, with dilation of the ureter and pelvis of the kidney. In this case, the bladder, ureter and pelvis with kidney cups are a single system, constantly filled with urine. The complete absence of emptying determines the need for catheterization of the bladder. In order to reduce the capacity of the bladder and reduce the volume of the ureter and pelvis for a week every month, we recommend installing a permanent catheter. The rest of the time, we use intermittent catheterization of the bladder. In addition, for any diseases with fever, as well as with an increase in the level of creatinine in the blood, a permanent catheter is also installed.

The main objective of treatment is to reduce the reflex closing activity of the sphincter (and pelvic floor muscles) and to make attempts to restore the detrusor tone and the closing function of the ureterovesical anastomosis. Active stimulating procedures on the bladder and the introduction of the most active anticholinesterase agent neostigmine methylsulfate ("proserin") are dangerous because of the risk, together with the restoration of detrusor activity, to get an increase in the degree of reflux. In the treatment, the following techniques are taken: courses of alpha-blockers, sinusoidal modulated currents in the antidystrophic mode on the bladder, nicotinic acid electrophoresis on L5-S2 segments, paraffin on the perineum, oral administration of ipidacrine, the use of metabolic therapy – preparations of magnesium and pyridoxine hydrochloride, L-carnitine. It should be noted that the treatment is carried out continuously, a monthly therapy regimen is compiled individually, the catheterization regimen is corrected depending on the appearance of the equivalent urge to urinate and the volume of residual urine. Every 3 months, a urodynamic examination is carried out for timely correction of disorders, with proper treatment, a slow decrease in the maximum cystometric capacity and a decrease in urethral closure pressure are detected. Together with a decrease in intraurethral pressure and the appearance of even a minimal detrusor tone, one can count on the appearance of an independent act of urination, according to uroflowmetry, this will be an obstructively interrupted urine flow, with the formation of a functionally obstructive variant over several years.

Atonic bladder and insufficiency of the urethral sphincter is a less dangerous urodynamic situation in terms of the development of complications from the upper urinary tract. With this variant of neurogenic bladder, we did not notice the formation of vesicoureteral reflux. This category of patients later develops nephrosclerosis. The bladder does not accumulate a large amount of urine due to its constant discharge from the urethra. During cystometry, from filling to 20-30 ml, the solution leaks past the catheter. The intravesical pressure is always low, and the urethral closure pressure is also low. The main task in this situation is to restore the tone and volume of the bladder and restore the retention function. For this purpose, courses of neostigmine methylsulfate, preparations of magnesium and pyridoxine hydrochloride, nicotinoyl-gamma-aminobutyric acid are used, alpha–blockers are used to improve the microcirculation of the bladder and urethra. Among the methods of physiotherapy, nicotinic acid electrophoresis is used on the sacrum, sinusoidal modulating currents in a stimulating mode on the perineum and bladder, physical therapy for training the pelvic floor and abdominal muscles, massage of the abdomen, thighs, buttocks, biofeedback therapy.

Patients with severe detrusor hypotension are treated with low-intensity laser energy, including a helium-neon (He-Ne) laser. The history of the therapeutic use of low-intensity laser energy in medicine and, in particular, in urology dates back to 1962. During this time, clinicians have become convinced of the effectiveness of low-intensity laser treatment of pathology associated with circulatory disorders. The energy of low-intensity lasers improves blood supply to parenchymal organs - kidneys, stimulates biological, immune, reparative processes, improves microcirculation.

Currently, the energy of low-intensity lasers is used to stimulate the contractility of elements of muscle structures, including detrusor. The stimulating effect of low-intensity lasers promotes the regeneration of contractile proteins actin and myosin, ensures the activation of cellular processes and the preservation of a sufficient number of intact mitochondria to generate adenosine triphosphate.

In this category of patients, He-Ne correction was performed with a 10mW laser at the location above the womb. A distinct positive effect on the volume velocity of the blood flow of the upper cystic artery was revealed according to Dopplerometry. The bubble reflex can be activated by laser exposure in 62% of observations. The rheography method reveals an increase in the speed of the rapid filling period – the blood filling of tissues improves, as well as vascular tone increases.

A drinking regime is used every 2 hours while awake and attempts to urinate after each intake of liquid. The correct vector of the chosen therapy clinically determines the appearance of an equivalent urge, the achievement of self-urination at least 20-70 ml intermittent jet, the appearance of a "dry" interval after urination for 60-90 minutes. Urodynamically, during repeated urethral profilometry, an increase in urethral closure pressure is recorded, and with cystometry, an increase in bladder capacity is recorded.

Given the combination of disorders of the bladder function and evacuation function of the distal colon, correction of pelvic functions should be carried out simultaneously. Constipation is corrected mainly by routine measures. Here, it is of great importance to teach parents various benefits in case of violation of emptying in a child. Despite the severe manifestations of colostasis, it is necessary to set the task of achieving the ideal variant of bowel emptying - in the morning, at the same time, at home. Before starting treatment, complete emptying of the intestines from fecal stones is necessary. For this purpose, enemas with saline solution are used, sometimes – a mechanical aid – the extraction of fecal stones from ampulla recti. After the initial complete bowel emptying, stimulating procedures are started to restore the passage. Immediately after waking up, they offer a cool drink – water or juice in a volume of at least 200 ml, after that – breakfast, then an attempt to visit the toilet. In the absence of an urge, the act of defecation is stimulated by rectal administration of a suppository with glycerin or with a small volume enema. Against the background of a laxative diet, lactulose intake and daily activities stimulating the function of the distal colon, a reflex for defecation is developed in the morning.

Conclusion

In neurology, spinal patients present the greatest difficulty for treatment, which consists in frequent recurrences of urinary tract infection, inadequate emptying of the bladder, the rapid appearance of complications from the upper urinary tract, leading to the development of chronic renal failure. At the same time, when there is a need for kidney transplantation in the terminal stage of chronic renal failure, children with neurogenic bladder undergoing periodic catheterization of the bladder may be limited in this possibility due to the risk of ascending infection [10]. The use of complex therapy of spinal neurogenic bladder can be supplemented with the use of antibacterial drugs based on the results of urine culture. Treatment regimens include the appointment of uroseptics for recurrent urinary tract infection and the presence of vesicoureteral reflux. Cephalosporin drugs of the 3rd generation are usually used (for oral administration – cefixime), as well as nitrofurans.

A large number of studies are conducted in neurology, but only a small part of them concerns spinal patients. Currently, there is no clear position concerning even the vector of further research work to improve the quality of life of this category of children. It is possible that neurosurgeons' research on the implantation of neurostimulators will be able to restore the function of pelvic organs, but this direction is still at the development stage. In this regard, any studies aimed at studying this condition are valuable for specialists to discuss the management tactics of this category of patients [11-19].

This study was performed using the Unique Scientific Unit (UNU) "Multicomponent software and hardware system for automated collection, storage, markup of research and clinical biomedical data, their unification and analysis based on Data Center with Artificial Intelligence technologies" (reg. number: 2075518).

References

[1] Blaas HGK, Eik-Nes SH, Isaksen CV. "The detection of spina bifida before 10 gestation weeks using two- and three- dimensional ultrasound." *Ultrasound Obstet. Gynecol.* 2000; 16 (1): 25-29.

[2] Trudell AS. "Diagnosis of spina bifida on ultrasound: always termination?" *Best Pract. Res. Clin. Obstet. Gynaecol.* 2014 Apr; 28 (3): 367-377.

[3] Ben-Sira L, Garel C, Malinger G, Constantini S. "Prenatal diagnosis of spinal dysraphism." *Childs Nerv. Syst.* 2013 Sep; 29 (9): 1541-1552.

[4] *Myelodysplasia in children (organization and provision of specialized medical care): A guide for doctors.* Rozinov VM., ed. Moscow: "Predanie," 2017: 220. (in Russ.)

[5] Deryugina LA. Disorders of the urodynamics of the lower urinary tract in fetuses. *Detskaya hirurgiya [Pediatric surgery].* 2007; 3: 30-34. (in Russ.).

[6] Vishnevskij EL. "*Overactive bladder.*" Materials of the Plenum of the Board of the Russian Society of Urologists, 2005, Tyumen, pp 322–343. (in Russ.).

[7] Madersbaher H. The various types of neurogenic bladder disfunction: an update of current therapeutic conception. *Paraplegia.* 1990 May; 28 (4): 217-229.

[8] Olandoski KP, Kolch V, Trigo-Rocha FE. Renal function in children with congenital neurogenic bladder. *Clinics.* 2011; 66 (2): 189-195.

[9] Nikitin SS. "Combined pelvic organ dysfunction in children." *Medicinskij akademicheskij zhurnal [Medical academic journal].* 2011; 1: 75–80. (in Russ.).

[10] Larijani FJ, Moghtaderi M, Hajizadeh N, Assadi F. Preventing kidney injury in children with neurogenic bladder dysfunction. *J. Prev. Med.* 2013 Dec; 4 (12): 1359-1364.

[11] Guseva NB., Nikitin SS. "Neurophysiological aspects of urinary disorders of inorganic genesis in children, basic principles of diagnosis and treatment." *Pediatriya [Pediatrics].* 2017; 96 (5):137-144 (in Russ.).

[12] Bavani AG, Hanafi MG, Sarkarian M. An investigation into the sensitivity of shear wave ultrasound elastography to measure the anterior bladder wall pressure in patients with neurogenic bladder. *J. Family Med. Prim. Care.* 2019 Apr; 8 (4): 1342-1346.

[13] Thomas DT, Yener S, Kalyoncu A, Uluc K, Bayri Y, Dagcinar A, Dagli T, Tugtepe H. Somatosensory evoked potentials as a screening tool for diagnosis of spinal pathologies in children with treatment refractory overactive bladder. *J. Childs Nerv. Syst.* 2017 Aug; 33 (8): 1327-1333.

[14] Borch L, Rittig S, Kamperis K, Mahler B, Djurhuus JC, Hagstroem S. No immediate effect on urodynamic parameters during transcutaneous electrical nerve stimulation (TENS) in children with overactive bladder and daytime incontinence-A randomized, double-blind, placebo-controlled study. *Neurourol. Urodyn.* 2017 Sep; 36 (7): 1788-1795.

[15] Kroll P, Gajewska E, Zachwieja J, Sobieska M, Mańkowski P. An Evaluation of the Efficacy of Selective Alpha-Blockers in the Treatment of Children with Neurogenic Bladder Dysfunction--Preliminary Findings. *Int. J. Environ. Res. Public Health.* 2016 Mar 15; 13 (3): 130-133.

[16] Lee B, Featherstone N, Nagappan P, McCarthy L, O'Toole S. British Association of Paediatric Urologists consensus statement on the management of the neuropathic bladder. *J. Pediatr. Urol.* 2016 Apr; 12 (2): 76-87.
[17] Moeller Joensson I, Hagstroem S, Siggaard C, Bower W, Djurhuus JC, Krogh K. Transcutaneous Electrical Nerve Stimulation Increases Rectal Activity in Children. *J. Pediatr. Gastroenterol. Nutr.* 2015 Jul; 61 (1): 80-84.
[18] Korzeniecka-Kozerska A, Zawada BO, Skutnik JM, Wasilewska A. The assessment of thiol status in children with neurogenic bladder caused by meningomyelocele. *Urol. J.* 2014 May 6; 11 (2): 1400-1405.
[19] Şekerci ÇA, Işbilen B, Işman F, Akbal C, Şimşek F, Tarcan T. Urinary NGF, TGF-β1, TIMP-2 and bladder wall thickness predict neurourological findings in children with myelodysplasia. *J. Urol.* 2014 Jan; 191 (1): 199-205.

Chapter 4

Vesicoureteral Reflux in a Child with Combined Pelvic Organ Dysfunction: A Clinical Observation

Sergei Nikitin[1,2,*], MD
Natalia Guseva[3-5], MD
Svetlana Kononova[6]
and Vadim Nikitin[1]

[1]Medical institute, Petrozavodsk State University, Petrozavodsk, Russia
[2]Children's Republican Hospital named after I. N. Grigovich, Petrozavodsk, Russia
[3]Russian Medical Academy of Continuous Professional Education, Moscow, Russia
[4]Department of Pediatric Surgery Pirogov Medical University, Moscow, Russia
[5]Moscow Voiding Dysfunction Center Moscow Paediatric Speransky Hospital No. 9, Moscow, Russia
[6]Department of Pediatrics and Pediatric Surgery, Medical Institute of PetrSU, Petrozavodsk, Russia

Abstract

Combined pelvic organ dysfunction in children is a new term that is just beginning to be used as a diagnosis in Russian pediatric practice. Until now, a large number of pediatricians and narrower specialists mistakenly consider violations of the function of the lower urinary tract and rectum in isolation from each other, without receiving the desired treatment results. Such a "separate," systemic-organ tactic, when a urologist is engaged in a violation of voiding, and a violation of the function of the rectum remains without medical attention or is transferred to the

---

* Correesponsing Author's Email: ssnikitin@yandex.ru.

In: Vesicoureteral Reflux
Editor: Garry M. Morones
ISBN: 979-8-89113-444-7
© 2024 Nova Science Publishers, Inc.

supervision of a gastroenterologist, not only does not lead to the recovery of the patient, but also delays the treatment process, contributes to the development of complications – vesicoureteral reflux, chronic kidney disease, megacolon, "fecal" intoxication with anemia. Moreover, often the patients themselves and their parents tend to talk about one problem – a violation of voiding or constipation – about the problem that at this stage worsens the quality of life of the patient to a greater extent. In this regard, it is very important to thoroughly collect anamnesis and complex treatment of combined pelvic organ dysfunction when they are detected.

The most common complication of neurogenic dysfunctions of the lower urinary tract, occurring in more than half of children with such disorders, is vesicoureteral reflux. The most reliable way to diagnose reflux is miction cystography, which allows, moreover, to establish its degree. Treatment of secondary vesicoureteral reflux begins with regimen-corrective measures. If they are ineffective, they switch to physiotherapy and drug treatment methods. In the case of recurrent urinary tract infections, the appointment of antibacterial therapy for up to several months is considered justified. If conservative methods of treatment are ineffective, they proceed to surgical correction – they begin with endoscopic plastic surgery of the ureter's mouth, and after two unsuccessful attempts they proceed to a more extensive surgical technique – the creation of a neoureterocystoanastomosis.

Unidirectional treatment – only neurogenic dysfunction of the bladder or only dysfunction of the colon and rectum usually do not bring lasting results. Only combined treatment makes it possible to adequately correct pelvic functions and exclude possible complications.

This article presents a clinical observation – the medical history of a 6-year-old girl with combined pelvic organ dysfunction, which was manifested by hyperactive bladder syndrome and constipation. The features of this clinical observation were several complicating factors: the presence of 2-sided vesicoureteral reflux of the 3rd degree with extremely high detrusor activity, the inability to treat a child with M-cholinoblockers due to a serious allergic reaction to this group of drugs, as well as persistent non-compliance at home with recommendations concerning the restoration of colon function with the support of a district pediatrician. Nevertheless, persistent cognitive and behavioral therapy made it possible to take control of the function of the pelvic organs and stop vesicoureteral reflux without any interventions and the use of antimuscarinic agents.

Keywords: children, combined dysfunction of the pelvic organs, overactive bladder, constipation, vesicoureteral reflux

Introduction

Combined pelvic organ dysfunction is a serious medical and social problem that reduces the quality of life of patients and their environment [1]. This concept implies a simultaneous violation of voiding and evacuation function of the colon. The frequency of occurrence of combined pelvic disorders is about 500 observations per 10,000 children. Violation of voiding - as a rule, these are manifestations of various variants of neurogenic dysfunctions of the bladder (overactive, underactive bladder, detrusor-sphincter dissinergia, stress incontinence and other variants), and violation of the function of the colon and rectum in the form of paradoxical encopresis, are a manifestation, to a greater extent, of pathology of inorganic genesis. In literary sources, a separate description of these dysfunctions is more common. Standard therapy, which is prescribed for bladder dysfunction or constipation, cannot claim success with combined pelvic organ dysfunction due to isolated effects only on the colon or bladder, it is an integrated approach to solving the problem that is important [2-3].

In the absence of timely and comprehensive correction of pelvic dysfunction, vesicoureteral reflux, developing against the background of neurogenic dysfunctions of the lower urinary tract, and colostasis can lead to recurrent urinary tract infections, the formation of chronic kidney disease, megacolon and "fecal" intoxication with anemia [3-4].

Secondary vesicoureteral reflux is the most common complication of lower urinary tract dysfunctions - according to some data, the prevalence of reflux in children with such disorders is 40-60%. At the same time, the development of vesicoureteral reflux against the background of urodynamic disorders of the lower urinary tract correlates with a higher probability of development and severity of reflux nephropathy than in the primary variant [5].

According to Morozov S. L. et al., neurogenic bladder dysfunctions of the overreflective type in the etiology of vesicoureteral reflux in children occupy up to 20% of cases. With this type of pathology, spontaneous contractions of the detrusor are recorded during the filling phase of the bladder. Such contractions lead to pronounced hypertrophy of the bladder wall, as a result of which the closing function of the ureterovesical anastomosis decreases (pseudodiverticles are formed, the bladder thickens), and vesicoureteral reflux occurs [6].

Urodynamic studies are mandatory for patients with neurogenic dysfunctions of the lower urinary tract and suspected vesicoureteral reflux:

uroflowmetry, urethral profilometry, retrograde cystometry, in some cases ureterovesical anastomosis profilometry, etc. The most universal urodynamic study is uroflowmetry. During this study, the volume and time of voiding are recorded. Based on these data, a uroflowmetric curve is formed – the dependence of the volumetric flow rate (ml/s) on time. A domed curve is considered normal, in the presence of pathologies, a curve in the form of "staccato", "plateau", obstructive-interrupted urination, rapid flow, etc., are recorded. The data of the uroflowmetric study in combination with the clinical picture allow us to establish the type of neurogenic dysfunction [5, 7]. Additional recording of the electrical activity of the pelvic floor muscles during uroflowmetry makes it possible to diagnose detrusor-sphincter dissinergia with greater accuracy [8].

Miction cystography is the most reliable way to diagnose vesicoureteral reflux. During this study, an X-ray contrast agent is injected into the bladder through a catheter in the supine position of the child. The introduction is carried out under the control of an electron-optical converter until the urge to urinate appears or until the age-related physiological capacity of the bladder is reached. After that, two snapshots are taken: the first is immediately after the introduction of a contrast agent, it allows you to detect passive reflux that occurs during the filling phase; the second is during voiding, it allows you to detect active reflux that occurs during the emptying phase. It should be noted that active reflux may go unnoticed if the child is unable to urinate during the study [5, 9-10].

The treatment of vesicoureteral reflux is aimed at eliminating its cause. In the case of secondary reflux, in most cases - for the correction of neurogenic dysfunction of the bladder. If vesicoureteral reflux is detected against the background of neurogenic bladder dysfunction, treatment begins with behavioral therapy. It consists in the formation of adequate hydration and stimulation of the function of emptying the bladder. To do this, the child is offered to drink every 2 hours during the waking period and empty the bladder after each intake of fluid. The emptying of the rectum is controlled [11-12].

With recurrent pyelonephritis against the background of vesicoureteral reflux, antibacterial therapy is prescribed. The most widely used cephalosporin antibiotics of the 3rd generation and nitrofurans. When identifying flora producing extended-spectrum beta-lactamases, the selection of the drug is carried out based on the results of urine culture with the determination of sensitivity to antibiotics. With frequently recurrent urinary tract infections, the appointment of prolonged antibiotic therapy for a period of several months is considered justified [9].

For the treatment of neurogenic bladder dysfunctions, physiotherapy methods are actively used. Their popularity is explained by the impact on all pathogenetic links of such disorders, noninvasiveness, absence of complications and the possibility of use in young children [13].

The method of dynamic electroneurostimulation is used, its effect leads to an increase in the effective volume of the bladder, a decrease in intravesical pressure [14].

The system of detrusor-stabilizing reflexes is effectively affected by the method of anal stimulation with interference and sinusoidal simulated currents. Such currents have low energy and can be applied purposefully to deeply located organs [14]. The method is also effective in the treatment of combined pelvic organ dysfunction, provided that such disorders occur against the background of immaturity of vegetative innervation - clinically, the improvement is manifested in the form of a decrease in episodes of encopresis and manifestations of lower urinary tract dysfunction [15].

To improve the trophic detrusor and eliminate metabolic disorders in its wall, phono- and electrophoresis is used on the bladder area of drugs that improve microcirculation (for example, nicotinic acid and euphyllin). Laser infrared radiation to the bladder area and the sacral spine normalizes the act of urination and detrusor tone - according to retrograde cystometry, the sensitivity threshold and reflex excitability of the bladder are normalized, its trophic improves. The method of heat treatment using mud, paraffin and ozokerite applications is widely used. The positive effect is associated with thermal, compression and chemical effects on the bladder area [14].

The method of biofeedback has gained the greatest popularity. During the procedure, the child is shown an interactive video sequence on the screen, with which he can interact by changing the activity of the pelvic floor muscles and the sphincter apparatus. During biofeedback therapy, the equipment only registers biological signals of the body, but does not affect the child directly. The main objective of this method is to teach the child self–regulation and self-control of the pelvic floor muscles and the sphincter apparatus. The use of the method in hyperactive bladder helps to reduce the level of residual urine, prevent an increase in intra-abdominal pressure, and with combined violations of the pelvic organs, a positive effect is also noted on the function of the rectum [6, 14, 16].

Physiotherapeutic methods, to increase their effectiveness, are used in conjunction with physical therapy and massage, aimed at strengthening the muscles of the pelvic floor and anterior abdominal wall [14].

Drug treatment of overactive bladder, as a pathology most often responsible for the development of vesicoureteral reflux, is usually started with the appointment of M-cholinoblockers. The mechanism of action is based on the blockade of muscarinic holinoreceptors of detrusor, this reduces its sensitivity to acetylcholine and levels the manifestations of overactivity – the intravesical pressure decreases and the capacity of the bladder increases, the accumulative function is restored. Most often, all drugs in this group are prescribed orally, but it is also possible to use electrophoresis on the bladder area. When detrusor-sphincter dissinergia is detected, drugs of the alpha-blockers group (doxazosin, tamzulosin) are prescribed [7].

If the conservative treatment of secondary vesicoureteral reflux is ineffective, it is switched to its surgical correction. Two methods of surgical treatment are most often used: endoscopic modeling of the ureteral mouth and Cohen neoimplantation of the ureter. The endoscopic method of treatment consists in bringing the volume-forming substance under the mucous membrane of the intramural ureter during cystoscopy [9, 17]. Thus, a dense base is created below the ureteral lumen, thereby lengthening its submucosal section. During miction, intravesical pressure increases, and the upper wall of the ureter presses against the lower one, which lies on a dense base, preventing retrograde urine discharge – this improves the antireflux function of the vesicoureteral segment [18].

Three methods of endoscopic reflux correction are widely used [19]:

- STING (Subureteral Transurethral Injection) – the introduction of a volume-forming drug directly below the mouth of the ureter
- HIT1 (Hydrodistance Implantation Technique 1) – the introduction of a volumizing drug only into the distal part of the intramural ureter
- HIT2 (Hydrodistance Implantation Technique 2) - the introduction of a volumizing drug into both the distal and proximal parts of the intramural ureter

The choice of endoscopic correction technique is based on the possibility of expanding the ureter's mouth with fluid flow during cystoscopy, depending on this, several degrees of hydrodilation are distinguished [20]:

1) H0 – when trying to hydrodilate, the mouth of the ureter does not open

2) H1 – the mouth of the ureter opens slightly during hydrodilation, it is impossible to get a cystoscope into the ureter
3) H2 – the mouth of the ureter opens when hydrodilation is attempted, it is possible to start a cystoscope only in the intramural part of the ureter
4) H3 – the mouth of the ureter opens when hydrodilation is attempted, a full-fledged ureteroscopy is possible

If the ureteral mouth is detected with a degree of hydrodilation H0 and H1, endoscopic correction can only be performed using the STING technique. When detecting the degree of hydrodilation of H2 and H3, it is possible to use any of the techniques [19].

The issue of choosing the most effective volumizing drug is debatable. Such a drug must meet all safety requirements (do not migrate in a short time and do not give a pronounced granulomatous reaction) and give the highest possible frequency of relief of reflux when using it. Currently, the following drugs are most widely used: collagen (of animal origin), DAM+ (a Russian-made drug consisting of a three-dimensional polyacrylamide mesh polymer, purified water and silver ions), urodex (an analog of the drug "Deflux" used in Russia and Europe, consisting of dextranomer microspheres and hyaluronic acid) and vantris (a preparation consisting of polyacrylate-poly-alcohol copolymer particles immersed in a 40% glycerol solution). Studies comparing the effectiveness of these substances have shown the greatest effectiveness of two of them – urodex and vantris. However, given the low density of urodex and its tendency to retrograde needle extrusion during administration, vantris, which has a denser consistency, is most often preferred [19, 21].

Another option for surgical treatment of vesicoureteral reflux is neoimplantation of the ureter. The most common method of such an operation according to Cohen: an incision of the anterior abdominal wall and a cystotomy is performed, the mouth of the ureter is excised and placed in the formed submucosal tunnel. The distal end of the ureter is sewn to the wall of the bladder, the defect in it is sutured. The vesicoscopic modification of Cohen's operation is gaining popularity: the bladder is filled with carbon dioxide; the pressure is maintained at 12 mmHg. For example, an optical trocar (6 mm) is installed approximately in the middle of the distance from the pubic joint to the navel, the other two (for instruments) are installed transrectally at the same distance from the first. The ureter is excised by an acute method, then a submucosal tunnel is formed in the bladder, and the ureter is carried into it.

The bladder defect is sutured, and the distal end of the ureter is sutured to the bladder wall [17, 22].

Currently, the choice of surgical treatment of vesicoureteral reflux increasingly falls on the endoscopic method of correction. Until recently, correction of low-grade vesicoureteral reflux (1-3) was performed using the endoscopic method, proceeding to the operation to form a neoureterocystoanastomosis after 2 unsuccessful attempts, and high-grade reflux forced doctors to immediately proceed to a more traumatic surgical intervention. Now, in order to prevent unnecessary traumatization of patients, it is proposed to begin surgical treatment of vesicoureteral reflux of all degrees with endoscopic correction, and to proceed to Cohen's operation only after two unsuccessful attempts of minimally invasive intervention. Thus, in a study conducted by Zorkin S. N. et al., the effectiveness of endoscopic correction of reflux of 4-5 degrees was studied. After the first injection of the volume-forming substance, the method proved to be effective (complete relief of reflux or its reduction to 1 degree) in 68.7% of cases. Among the remaining children, after the second summing up of the volume-forming substances, the treatment was effective for 48.9% of patients. Patients for whom endoscopic correction proved ineffective were operated according to Cohen's or Politano-Leatbetter's methods. Thus, the minimally invasive technique of surgical correction of reflux avoids unnecessary traumatization of patients with results not much inferior to extensive surgical technique [23].

Endoscopic plastic surgery of the ureteral mouth is also recognized as a more effective alternative to the appointment of permanent antibiotic therapy in comparison with the number of episodes of febrile urinary tract infections [9, 17].

Neurogenic bladder dysfunctions in 40-45% of cases are combined with disorders of rectal function, which are clinically manifested by constipation and encopresis. In most cases, constipation, which patients treat, is of a functional nature. The mechanism of development of functional constipation is largely similar to that of neurogenic bladder dysfunctions – vascular spasm and ischemia lead to hyperactivation of alpha-adrenergic receptors and impaired rectal function. Prolonged colostasis with the formation of fecal stones gradually transforms the colon and rectum into a megacolon and megarectum. [24].

During the initial treatment of parents with children, it is often problematic to establish that pelvic organ dysfunction is combined. Often patients complain either only of constipation and encopresis, or of dysfunction of the lower urinary tract. Moreover, often children and their parents do not even notice the second side of the violations, since its manifestations are subclinical in nature. Therefore, when treating patients with complaints of pelvic organ dysfunction, a targeted and thorough collection of anamnesis is important [24].

The distal parts of the urinary system and the gastrointestinal tract are connected by the pelvic diaphragm, are located close to each other in the pelvic cavity and are subject to mutual interference with impaired function. Pelvic organs perform similar functions (accumulation, retention, excretion), and have common sources of innervation and blood supply. Because of this, violations occurring simultaneously in both of these systems negatively affect each other. For the same reason, it is the functional approach that is important here, and not the system-organ approach, i.e., comprehensive diagnosis and treatment of dysfunctions of related organ systems [16].

This publication presents a clinical case that demonstrates the features of examination and treatment of a child who has combined pelvic organ dysfunction – overactive bladder, constipation during the week, encopresis and bilateral vesicoureteral reflux of the 3rd degree. The situation was complicated by the inability to prescribe an M-cholinoblocker - the drug of choice for relieving detrusor overactivity - due to the presence of a pronounced allergic reaction to this group of drugs in a child [7]. It is absolutely mandatory to have a full understanding between the doctor and parents in connection with the need for constant monitoring of the function of the pelvic organs.

Girl R. 6 years old, sent to a surgical hospital as planned for examination (informed parental consent for hospitalization, all methods of examination and treatment received) due to complaints of imperative urinary incontinence during the daytime, enuresis 2 times a night from an early age. There were no manifestations of urinary tract infection, urine tests were always within normal limits. A pronounced allergic reaction to M-cholinoblockers in the form of shortness of breath attacks did not allow prescribing drugs of this group. In addition, the child has constipation – the urge to defecate is present, the stool is independent, 1 time a week, large diameter, rocky density. At the same time, parents did not focus on constipation, the fact of their presence was established during the targeted collection of anamnesis about the state of pelvic organ function. Parents found it difficult to answer the question about the prescription of manifestations of colostasis, at home this issue was not controlled for several years. Upon admission, the child's condition is satisfactory. Proper physique, satisfactory nutrition. The skin is pale pink and dry. The mucous membranes are clean. In the lungs, vesicular respiration is carried out in all departments, the number of breaths is 20 per minute. The heart tones are rhythmic, the number of heartbeats is 90 per minute. The abdomen is not swollen, symmetrical, participates in the act of breathing. When palpated, it is soft, accessible to deep examination, painless in all departments. Fecal stones are determined in the descending part of the colon. Intestinal motility is uniformly weakened. The analysis of the urination diary revealed 14-27 urinations per day, volumes from 5 to 85 ml. The volume of fluid that the child received was less than 500 ml per day.

According to the results of ultrasound examination of the abdominal cavity and organs of the urinary system, the presence of bilateral pyeloectasia (anterior-posterior diameter 12-14 mm), a small volume of the bladder and a thickening of its wall to 6 mm was determined. Scanning of the colon revealed the expansion of its loops. Biochemical blood test – within normal limits (total protein 76 g\l, albumin 38 g\l, creatinine 57 mkmol\l, urea 4 mmol\l, potassium 3.6 mmol\l, sodium 138 mmol\l, bilirubin 13 mkmol\l). General urine analysis – without pathology: relative density 1022, pH 5.5, protein 0, glucose 0, erythrocytes, leukocytes 0. Urine culture is sterile.

A urodynamic study was conducted. According to the results of uroflowmetry (monitoring), obstructive-interrupted urination is recorded. Cystometry: 70 ml of saline solution was injected into the bladder while lying down. During the study, non-inhibited contractions of the detrusor with high pressure (up to 85 cm H2O) are recorded. Urethral profilometry – the closure function is not impaired. Conclusion. Overactive bladder with pronounced detrusor activity.

Mictional cystourethrography was performed – 2-sided vesicoureteral reflux of the 3rd degree was detected.

Irrigation with barium sulfate contrast was performed, megacolon of the 2nd degree was detected, emptying was adequate.

A rheopelviography was performed – a decrease in blood filling of the anterior parts of the pelvis was revealed (according to the systolic amplitude of the pulse wave and the maximum speed of the rapid filling period).

In the department, hydrocolonotherapy was performed for colostasis, a forced drinking regime was started - every 2 hours 200 ml per day – 1800-2000 ml. Lactulose is prescribed for 20 ml in the morning. Methods of physiotherapy were used – biofeedback therapy, synsoidal modulating currents on the perineum, acupuncture, paraffin therapy on the bladder. Taking into account the impossibility of prescribing M-cholinoblockers due to an allergic reaction and a decrease in the level of blood filling in the projection of the pelvis, alpha-blockers were prescribed (doxazosin in a small dose - 0.25 mg at night – for 3 months). Against this background, daily bowel emptying appeared, the volume of urination increased slightly – up to 50-120 ml, the nature of the uroflowmetric curve improved, which began to correspond to the functionally obstructive variant.

Upon discharge, the diagnosis is formulated as follows: overactive bladder with detrusor activity. Bilateral vesicoureteral reflux of the 3rd degree. Secondary chronic pyelonephritis, latent course, without impaired renal function. At home, it is recommended to monitor defecation, teach to empty at the same time, in the morning - to develop a reflex for defecation. Stimulation of morning defecation by taking cool liquid on an empty stomach, correction of nutrition, use of laxatives if necessary.

To correct enuresis, it is recommended to use alarm-therapy.

After discharge from the hospital, the recommendations were implemented only partially and only during the first week after discharge. Further, the parents explained that the girl herself could not control the issues of drinking, urination and defecation, and it was not possible to find time for parental control. The drinking regime was again restricted. Constipation reappeared up to 6-7 days, against which the manifestations of imperative urination syndrome became more frequent. It should be noted that the district pediatrician did not support the idea of the need for daily bowel movement, considering the individual rhythm of defecation in a child to be physiological. In this regard, an interim examination after 8 months showed similar results as in the first hospitalization. Vesicoureteral reflux from 2 sides of the 3rd degree and pronounced detrusor activity persisted. According to the results of biochemical blood tests, renal dysfunction was not detected.

A certain turning point in the next conversation with parents about the need to control the function of the pelvic organs of the child was the appearance of an encopresis on the 4-5 day constipation, which began to create additional problems – the smell, the need to change clothes, psychological problems. At this stage, after the next elimination of colostasis, the child's parents began to follow all our recommendations with entries in the diary of voiding and defecation of the dynamics of pelvic organ function. If in the first month of treatment, a hypertensive enema had to be performed every other day, then at the 6th month, enemas were not required even once, it was only necessary to remind the child about visiting the toilet in the morning. Against the background of regular bowel emptying for 6 months, the volume of the bladder was 80-200 ml, the number of voidings per day corresponded to the recommended one – every 2 hours during the waking period. The use of a urinary alarm clock allowed us to reduce the frequency of enuresis to 1 time per week. Another examination showed stabilization of detrusor function according to cystometry data – maladaptation was stopped, the maximum cystometric capacity was 350 ml. Miction cystography was performed – no reflux was detected. Ultrasound of the bladder – the wall is 3 mm.

The above clinical observation is combined violations of pelvic functions, with 2–sided vesicoureteral reflux of the 3rd degree, extremely pronounced detrusor overactivity and the inability to prescribe oxybutynin hydrochloride, trospium chloride, and other M-cholinoblockers due to an allergic reaction, using cognitive and behavioral techniques - regimen methods that change the drinking stereotype and attitude the patient and parents to the function of excretion, allowed to solve the problem of urinary incontinence, constipation with encopresis, to stop vesicoureteral reflux and detrusor overactivity. This example indicates the need for parental control and control of a pediatrician in case of pelvic organ dysfunction in children. The effectiveness of treatment of children with combined pelvic dysfunction is possible only if the simultaneous correction of the function of voiding and defecation.

Conclusion

Combined pelvic organ dysfunction is a problem that requires comprehensive diagnosis and treatment. When treating patients with complaints of urination disorders or constipation and encopresis, the doctor should find out whether these complaints have a second side. The most common complication of neurogenic dysfunctions of the lower urinary tract, as an element of combined disorders, is vesicoureteral reflux. Treatment of secondary vesicoureteral reflux, which has arisen against the background of combined pelvic organ disorders, begins with routine corrective measures - ensuring adequate hydration, monitoring the emptying of the bladder and rectum. With the ineffectiveness of behavioral measures, drug treatment is transferred, which is prescribed depending on the type of neurogenic dysfunction. Physiotherapeutic measures are also used, among which the methods of anal stimulation and biofeedback have the greatest effectiveness in combined disorders of the pelvic organs. If conservative therapy is ineffective, they switch to surgical methods of correction of reflux – they begin with endoscopic plastic surgery of the ureter's mouth, and after two unsuccessful attempts of minimally invasive treatment, they proceed to surgery for neoimplantation of the ureter.

The clinical case presented in the article demonstrates the features of diagnosis and treatment of a child with combined pelvic organ dysfunction. In this situation, due to the inability to prescribe M-cholinoblockers, treatment was limited to behavioral therapy and heat treatment. Nevertheless, these measures proved to be sufficient for the correction of combined pelvic organ dysfunction and associated vesicoureteral reflux.

This study was performed using the Unique Scientific Unit (UNU) "Multicomponent software and hardware system for automated collection, storage, markup of research and clinical biomedical data, their unification and analysis based on Data Center with Artificial Intelligence technologies" (reg. number: 2075518).

References

[1] Ignat'ev R. O., Guseva N. B., Nikitin S. S., Ry'zhov E. A., Fomenko O.Yu., Ponomareva T. N. "Opportunities to improve the quality of life of children with combined disorders of urination and defecation with the unification of diagnostic and treatment methods." *Detskaya xirurgiya.* [Pediatric Surgery] 2014; 5: 8–12. (in Russ.)

[2] Pisklakov A. V., Shevlyakov A. S. "Treatment of combined dysfunction of the pelvic organs in children." *Rossijskij vestnik perinatologii i pediatrii.* [Russian Bulletin of Perinatology and Pediatrics] 2012; 3: 96–99. (in Russ.)

[3] Nikitin S. S. "Disorders of neurohumoral regulation in combined dysfunction of the pelvic organs in children." *Doctor's thesis.* Moskva, 2016, 43 p. (in Russ.).

[4] Guseva N. B., Nikitin S. S. "Neurophysiological aspects of disorders urination of inorganic origin in children, the basic principles of diagnosis and treatment." *Pediatriya named after G N Speransky.* 2017; 96(5): 137–144. (in Russ.).

[5] Deryugina L. A. "Vesicoureteral reflux and its prenatal prognosis." *Pediatriya im. G.N. Speranskogo.* [Pediatriya named after G N Speransky] 2018; 97 (5): 14–19. doi: 10.24110/0031-403X2018-97-5-14-19. (in Russ.)

[6] Morozov S. L., Dlin V. V., Shabel'nikova E. I. "Biofeedback method in children with dysfunctional urination and overactive bladder, complicated by urinary incontinence, vesicoureteral reflux, nephropathy." *Praktika pediatra.* [Pediatrician practice] 2020; 2: 33–40. (in Russ.)

[7] Vorob'eva Yu. D., Sy't'kov V. V., Zokirov N.Z., Bushueva T. V., Yacyk S. P., Fedorova E.V. "Overactive bladder in children: new in diagnosis and treatment." *Rossijskij pediatricheskij zhurnal.* [Russian pediatric journal.] 2020; 23(5): 330-334. doi: 10.18821/1560-9561-2020-23-5-330-334. (in Russ.)

[8] Guseva N. B., Nikitin S.S., Ignat'ev R. O., Bozhendaev T. L. "Incomplete bladder emptying syndrome in children: spectrum of differential diagnosis." *Pediatriya named after G N Speransky.* 2019; 98 (5): 8-14. (in Russ.)

[9] Umalatova M. I., Lefitov G. M., Maxachev B. M. "Vesicoureteral reflux in children: clinic, diagnosis and approaches to therapy." *Sovremennaya nauka: aktual'ny'e*

problemy' teorii i praktiki. [Modern science: current problems of theory and practice] 2018; 6: 230-233. (in Russ.)

[10] Zorkin S. N., Shaxnovskij D. S., Turov F. O., Galuzinskaya A. T., D'yakonova E.Yu. "The effectiveness of endoscopic correction of high-grade vesicoureteral reflux in children." *Detskaya xirurgiya.* [Pediatric Surgery]. 2020; 24 (5): 292-296, doi: 10.18821/1560-9510-2020-24-5-292-296. (in Russ.)

[11] Novikova E. V. "Treatment and medical rehabilitation of children with overactive bladder." *Rossijskij vestnik detskoj xirurgii, anesteziologii i reanimatologii.* [Russian Bulletin of Pediatric Surgery, Anesthesiology and Reanimatology] 2018; 8 (4): 105-110, doi: 10.30946/2219-4061-2018-8-4-105-110. (in Russ.).

[12] Guseva N. B., Nikitin S. S., Varlamova T. V., Zaripova Yu.R. Vesicoureteral reflux in combination with dysfunction of the pelvic organs in an 8-year-old child. *Pediatriya named after G N Speransky.* 2020; 96 (5). (in Russ.)

[13] Novikova E. V., Xan M. A., Menovshhikova L. B. "The use of laser radiation and interference currents in the medical rehabilitation of children with neurogenic bladder dysfunction." *Voprosy' kurortologii, fizioterapii i lechebnoj fizicheskoj kul'tury*'[Questions of balneology, physiotherapy and physical therapy]. 2020; 98 (4): 71-76. doi: 10.38025/ 2078–1962– 2020–98–4–71–76. (in Russ.)

[14] Novikova E. V. "Treatment and medical rehabilitation of children with overactive bladder." *Rossijskij vestnik detskoj xirurgii, anesteziologii i reanimatologii.* [Russian Bulletin of Pediatric Surgery, Anesthesiology and Reanimatology] 2018; 8 (4): 105-110. doi: 10.30946/2219-4061-2018-8-4-105-110. (in Russ.)

[15] Pisklakov A. V., Shevlyakov A. S. "Treatment of combined dysfunction of the pelvic organs in children." *Rossijskij vestnik perinatologii i pediatrii.* [Russian Bulletin of Perinatology and Pediatrics.] 2012; 57(3): 96–99. (in Russ.)

[16] Moiseev A. B., Mironov A. A., Kol'be O. B., Vartapetova E. E., Polunina V. V., Al'-Sabunchi A. A., Polunin V. S., Buslaeva G. N. "Urination disorders and combined dysfunction of the pelvic organs in children: approaches to diagnosis, treatment and prevention." Vestnik Rossijskogo gosudarstvennogo medicinskogo universiteta. 2018; 5: 62–69. (in Russ.).

[17] Pirogov A. V., Sizonov V. V., Kogan M. I. "Comparative efficacy and safety of transurethral and vesicoscopic surgery for primary vesicoureteral reflux in children." *Vestnik urologii.* [Journal of Urology] 2020; 8: 58–68. (in Russ.)

[18] Burkin A. G., Yacyk S. P., Sharkov S. M., Rusakov A. A., Tin I. F. "Endoscopic treatment of vesicoureteral reflux in children." *Urologiya.* [Urology] 2014; 5: 102-106. (in Russ.)

[19] Barsegyan E. R., Zorkin S. N. "Comparative evaluation of the effectiveness of the use of various polymers in endoscopic correction of vesicoureteral reflux in children." *Detskaya xirurgiya.* [Pediatric Surgery] 2014; 18 (5): 4-8. (in Russ.)

[20] Cerwinka W. H., Scherz H. C., Kirsch A. J. Dynamic hydrodistention classification of the ureter and the double hit method to correct vesicoureteral reflux. *Archivos Espanoles de Urologia.* [Spanish Archives of Urology] 2008; 61 (8): 882-887.

[21] Abdullaev F. K., Kulaev V. D., Nikolaev V. V. "Dependence of the effectiveness of endoscopic treatment of primary vesicoureteral reflux on volume-forming material." *Urologiya.* [Urology] 2013; 2: 94-97. (in Russ.)

[22] Pirogov A. V., Sizonov V. V., Kogan M. I. "Experience of 157 vesicoscopic operations in children." *Urologiya* [Urology]. 2017; 6: 59-64. (in Russ.)
[23] Zorkin S. N., Shaxnovskij D. S., Turov F. O., Galuzinskaya A. T., D`yakonova E.Yu. "The effectiveness of endoscopic correction of high-grade vesicoureteral reflux in children." Detskaya xirurgiya. [Pediatric Surgery] 2020; 24 (5): 292-296. doi: 10.18821/1560-9510-2020-24-5-292-296. (in Russ.).
[24] Nikitin S. S. "Combined dysfunctions of the pelvic organs in children." Medicinskij akademicheskij zhurnal. 2011; 11(1): 75-80. (in Russ.)

About the Authors

Sergei Nikitin – MD, Professor of the Department of Pediatrics and Pediatric Surgery of the Medical Institute of the Petrozavodsk State University, Petrozavodsk; head of the surgical department and of the Center for Pediatric Urology, Andrology and Nephrology Children's Republican Hospital named after I. N. Grigovich, Petrozavodsk. ssnikitin@yandex.ru +7911-423-85-59 ORCID: 0000-0002-4920-1722.

Natalia Guseva – MD, Head of the Moscow Voiding Disfunction Center Moscow Paediatric Speransky Hospital No. 9, Chief Researcher of the Department of Pediatric Surgery Pirogov Medical University, Professor of the Department of Pediatrics of the Russian Medical Academy of Continuing Professional Education, Moscow. guseva-n-b@yandex.ru +7910-408-18-86 ORCID: 0000-0002-1583-1769.

Svetlana Kononova - senior lecturer of the Department of Pediatrics and Pediatric Surgery, Medical Institute of PetrSU, Petrozavodsk. svetlanakononova51@gmail.com +7909-571-87-76

Vadim Nikitin – student, Medical Institute of the Petrozavodsk State University, Petrozavodsk vadimnikitin11@yandex.ru +7911- 051-15-54 ORCID: 0000-0003-2236-0296.

Chapter 5

A Clinical Observation of the Conservative Treatment of Vesicoureteral Reflux on the Background of Detrusor-Sphincter Dyssinergia in an 8-Year-Old Child

Sergei Nikitin[1,2,*], **MD**
Natalia Guseva[3-5], **MD**
Svetlana Kononova[6]
and Vadim Nikitin[1]

[1]Medical institute, Petrozavodsk State University, Petrozavodsk, Russia
[2]Children's Republican Hospital named after I.N. Grigovich, Petrozavodsk, Russia
[3]Russian Medical Academy of Continuous Professional Education, Moscow, Russia
[4]Department of Pediatric Surgery Pirogov Medical University, Moscow, Russia
[5]Moscow Voiding Dysfunction Center Moscow Paediatric Speransky Hospital No. 9, Moscow, Russia
[6]Department of Pediatrics and Pediatric Surgery, Medical Institute of PetrSU, Petrozavodsk, Russia

Abstract

Vesicoureteral reflux is the most common form of urodynamic disorder in childhood, leading to the destruction of renal parenchyma as a result of kidney damage, the progression of chronic pyelonephritis and reflux nephropathy. Among the causes are anomalies in the development of the ureterovesical anastomosis, microbial-inflammatory process of the organs of the urinary system and bladder dysfunction of various genesis.

---

[*] Corresponding Author's Email: ssnikitin@yandex.ru.

In: Vesicoureteral Reflux
Editor: Garry M. Morones
ISBN: 979-8-89113-444-7
© 2024 Nova Science Publishers, Inc.

A combination of these reasons is often identified. One of the most significant variants of neurogenic bladder dysfunction in terms of the formation of vesicoureteral reflux is detrusor-sphincter dissinergia.

A clinical case of an 8-year-old patient with recurrent urinary tract infection is presented. It is known from the anamnesis that the child has a recurrent course of pyelonephritis for three years. About 2-3 times a year exacerbation of pyelonephritis with fever, and about once every two months – episodes of leukocyturia in urine tests. There are no clinically significant urination disorders. Episodes of pollakiuria up to 12 times a day were noted several times during periods of exacerbations of urinary system infection. There is no urinary incontinence, she also did not complain about painful urination. She was hospitalized for urgent indications 7 days after the onset of the disease with complaints of an increase in body temperature to 38.5 °C and abdominal pain with irradiation to the lumbar region. The child was diagnosed with "chronic pyelonephritis, exacerbation". Infusion therapy with solutions of crystalloids, antibacterial therapy with drugs of the cephalosporin group of the 3rd generation was carried out. Within 7 days, the manifestations of acute urinary system infection were stopped, the condition stabilized.

Immediately after the relief of acute inflammation, noninvasive diagnostic methods were performed. Invasive methods were carried out a month later to prevent the recurrence of pyelonephritis.

During uroflowmetry with simultaneous recording of electromyography of the pelvic floor muscles, signs of detrusor-sphincter dyssinergia were revealed. Subsequently, the presence of detrusor-sphincter dyssinergia was confirmed by the "pressure-flow" study. The method of rheopelviography revealed a decrease in the level of blood supply to the bladder. Miction cystography revealed vesicoureteral reflux on both sides of the second degree.

Based on the survey, it turned out that relapses of pyelonephritis were the end result of a chain of disorders in this child. The chain of disorders itself looks like this: detrusor-sphincter dyssinergia – reflux – pyelonephritis. It was decided to conduct a comprehensive conservative therapy, primarily aimed at the source of the disorders – detrusor-sphincter dyssinergia, as well as at the relief of urinary system infection. A treatment regimen is presented, which contains an alpha-adrenoblocker, uroseptics, physiotherapy methods and behavioral therapy.

After 6 months, miction cystography and uroflowmetry with recording of pelvic floor electromyography were repeated. No reflux was detected during mictional cystography. With uroflowmetry, a normal result was obtained, the manifestations of detrusor-sphincter dyssinergia were stopped. There were no changes in urine tests for 6 months.

In conclusion, the basics of the pathological physiology of detrusor-sphincter dyssinergia are presented. Detrusor-sphincter dyssinergia is the most common variant of functional infravesical obstruction. Unlike other variants of neurogenic bladder dysfunctions, with detrusor-sphincter dyssinergia, urinary incontinence is usually not detected and for this reason, this condition is often diagnosed only at the stage of complications, as in the described clinical observation. The main complications are vesicoureteral reflux and recurrent course of chronic pyelonephritis.

The pathogenesis of detrusor-sphincter dyssinergia is based on the following pathophysiological mechanisms. The activity of the urethral sphincter in detrusor-sphincter dyssinergia is due to a violation of the function of the miction center of the pons, which normally ensures the coordinated work of the detrusor and the external sphincter of the urethra, as well as the classical urination reflexes that ensure the emptying phase. The sequence of activation of 7-11 urination reflexes is disrupted: detrusor-urethral inhibitory, detrusor-sphincteral inhibitory, urethro-detrusor activating, urethro-sphincteral inhibitory and early activation of the 12th reflex – perineo-bulbar inhibitory. High detrusor pressure during voiding with an incompletely open urethral sphincter disrupts the closing function of the uretero-vesical anastomosis and develops vesicoureteral reflux with ascending urinary tract infection.

In connection with the above information, the correct treatment of detrusor-sphincter dyssinergia makes it possible to stop vesicoureteral reflux without surgical interventions.

Keywords: detrusor-sphincter dyssinergia, vesicoureteral reflux, pyelonephritis, children

Vesicoureteral reflux is the most common form of urodynamic disorders in childhood. Long-term vesicoureteral reflux leads to the destruction of the renal parenchyma as a result of kidney damage, the progression of chronic pyelonephritis and reflux nephropathy [1-4]. Vesicoureteral reflux occurs in 1% of children aged 0 to 15 years, of which bilateral lesion is up to 50.9%. In half of the patients, the degree of reflux varies from different sides [1]. The pathogenesis of vesicoureteral reflux is very complex and many issues remain debatable. Among the causes are anomalies in the development of the ureterovesical anastomosis, microbial-inflammatory process of the organs of the urinary system and bladder dysfunction of various genesis. With vesicoureteral reflux, a combination of these factors is more often diagnosed. Malformations of the lower urinary tract are often combined with an anomaly of kidney development. This combination has been called "CAKUT syndrome" (genital anomalies of kidney and urinary tract) [5, 6]. Among kidney defects in children with vesicoureteral reflux, doubling and hypoplasia are more common. The introduction of ultrasound screening into obstetric and pediatric practice has significantly increased the early detection of abnormalities in the development of the urinary system. In children with antenatal dilation of the pelvis, vesicoureteral reflux occurs in 15-38% of cases [7]. The existence of hereditary vesicoureteral reflux has been established, which is caused by a mutation of one or more genes encoding extracellular protein components of the ureterovesical anastomosis and other elements of the urinary system. Genetically determined vesicoureteral reflux is characteristic of individuals with hereditary connective tissue dysplasia [8-10]. Among all children, vesicoureteral reflux is detected in more than 50% of cases before the age of 1 year. For the diagnosis of reflux, miction cystography is used – a method of X-ray contrast examination of the bladder and urethra. Indications for cystography are recurrent infection of the urinary system, as well as changes detected by ultrasound examination of the organs of the urinary system (kidney anomaly, dilatation of the renal pelvis and ureters, the presence of residual urine, etc.), urinary incontinence and other various urination disorders. Despite the fact that significant malformations of the organs of the urinary system are detected by ultrasound examination in the perinatal period, anomalies such as hypoplasia and doubling of the kidney can manifest themselves only by size asymmetry and often remain without proper observation for a number of years. In these cases, in the presence of vesicoureteral reflux, its long-term existence contributes to the development and progression of reflux nephropathy [1-4]. Considering that the management tactics of children with vesicoureteral reflux is ambiguous and controversial on a number of issues of diagnosis and treatment, we present a clinical observation of a patient with vesicoureteral reflux.

In the center of urology of the Children's Republican Hospital of the city of Petrozavodsk, a girl P.M. 8 years old was treated. She was hospitalized for urgent indications 7 days after the onset of the disease with complaints of an increase in body temperature to 38.5 ºC and abdominal pain with irradiation to the lumbar region. The provoking factor was hypothermia – bathing in an open pond in cool weather. It is known from the anamnesis that the child has a recurrent course of pyelonephritis for three years. About 2-3 times a year exacerbations of pyelonephritis with fever, and about once every two months – episodes of leukocyturia in urine tests. There are no clinically significant urination disorders. Episodes of pollakiuria up to 12 times a day were noted several times during periods of exacerbations of urinary system infection.

There is no urinary incontinence, she also did not complain about painful urination.

The hereditary factor is burdened – the child's mother has chronic pyelonephritis against the background of an overactive bladder since childhood. At the age of 6, the girl's mother underwent surgery for vesicoureteral reflux on the right (Cohen neoimplantation of the ureter).

Upon admission, she was examined by a surgeon – surgical pathology of the abdominal organs is excluded. On examination, there was a positive symptom of pounding on the right lumbar region (Pasternatsky's symptom). Ultrasound examination of the kidneys and bladder was performed. Here is a detailed conclusion. The kidneys are located at the usual level. The dimensions of the right kidney are 85 ×30 mm, the left - 86 × 32 mm. The contours of the kidneys are clear, even. The cortical substance is clearly differentiated from the surrounding tissues. Cup-pelvic complexes are not expanded, signs of chronic inflammation are compaction of the walls of the pelvis and large cups, as well as a symptom characteristic of acute pyelonephritis - a double contour of the pelvis, formed against the background of edema. The bladder is oval in shape, the wall thickness is uneven – from 3 to 5 mm, the contents are homogeneous, foreign bodies are not detected, there is sediment at the bottom. The ureteral mouths and ureteral discharge are visualized. The terminal sections of the ureters are not visualized. Bladder volume up to 210 ml, residual volume 50 ml.

A laboratory examination of urine was performed: yellow, muddy, relative density 1030, pH 5.5. Protein 0.3 g \ l. Leukocytes 40-50 in the field of view, erythrocytes 10-15 in the field of view.

In clinical blood analysis, leukocytes 18×10^9 / l, erythrocytes 4.4×10^{12} / l, hemoglobin 115 g / l, platelets 552×10^9 /l, erythrocyte sedimentation rate 25 mm / hour.

In the biochemical analysis of blood, the level of C-reactive protein was increased to 65 mg /l, indicators of total protein and protein fractions, creatinine, urea, potassium, sodium, bilirubin, transaminases – without deviations from the norm.

The child was diagnosed with "chronic pyelonephritis, exacerbation." Infusion therapy with solutions of crystalloids, antibacterial therapy with drugs of the cephalosporin group of the 3rd generation was carried out. Within 7 days, the manifestations of acute urinary system infection were stopped, the condition stabilized. Positive dynamics was noted in laboratory parameters – normalization of the level of C-reactive protein, leukocytosis was stopped in clinical blood analysis, normalization of urine tests was noted. During the control ultrasound examination of the kidneys, the sign of acute pyelonephritis – the double contour of the pelvis was not determined.

After the stabilization of the condition, a decision was made to examine the child. Immediately after the relief of acute inflammation, noninvasive diagnostic methods were performed. Invasive methods were carried out a month later to prevent the recurrence of pyelonephritis.

During uroflowmetry with simultaneous recording of electromyography of the pelvic floor muscles, signs of detrusor-sphincter dyssinergia were revealed. Normally, during voiding, an electromyographic pause from the pelvic floor muscles should be detected. No pelvic floor relaxation was registered in our patient during urination. There was only a 30% decrease in the tonic activity of the sphincter. In this regard, a rheopelviography was performed to assess the state of blood supply to the bladder. A decrease in the level of blood supply to the bladder was revealed – the indicator "systolic pulse wave amplitude" was reduced.

From the methods of invasive diagnosis, a month after the exacerbation of pyelonephritis, miction cystography and urodynamic examination were performed. Miction cystography revealed vesicoureteral reflux on both sides of the second degree (according to the classification of Heikkel-Poskulainen - throwing urine into the pelvis of the kidneys without dilation).

From the methods of studying urodynamics, taking into account the revealed uroflowmetry with electromyography of the pelvic floor, detrusor-sphincter dyssinergia, a "pressure-flow" study and urethral profilometry were performed. Let's present the protocol of urodynamic research.

The "pressure–flow" study was performed. During the filling phase, 180 ml of saline solution was injected into the bladder at a rate of 20 ml / min. During the filling process, normal detrusor and vesical pressure is recorded. There are no non-inhibited abbreviations. The first urge at a volume of 50 ml. During the filling phase, high-amplitude tonic activity is recorded from the pelvic floor muscles. During the emptying phase, an electromyographic pause from the pelvic floor muscles is not recorded. An obstructive type curve. Increase in detrusor pressure over 100 cmH_2O. There was an increase in abdominal pressure, the participation of the abdominal press during the act of urination. Urethral profilometry – catheter extraction at a rate of 2 mm/sec when fluid is supplied at a rate of 2 ml/min. The length of the sphincter is 1 cm. Closing pressure 135 cmH_2O. Conclusion of the study: detrusor-sphincter dyssinergia.

Taking into account the information received, the diagnosis was made: "neurogenic dysfunction of the bladder – detrusor-sphincter dyssinergia.

Vesicoureteral reflux on both sides of the second degree. Secondary chronic pyelonephritis, recurrent course, without renal failure."

Thus, relapses of pyelonephritis were the end result of a chain of disorders in this child. The chain of disorders itself looks like this: detrusor-sphincter dyssinergia – reflux – pyelonephritis. In this situation, we considered it inappropriate to perform endoscopic correction of vesicoureteral reflux. We believe that it made no sense to influence reflux without treatment of neurogenic bladder dysfunction. It also didn't make sense to treat only pyelonephritis with antibiotics. Therefore, it was decided to conduct complex therapy, primarily aimed at the source of disorders – detrusor-sphincter dyssinergia.

First of all, the regime of drinking and urination was formed. The drinking regime consisted in taking 200 ml of liquid every 2 hours from 7 a.m. to 7 p.m. For drinking, cranberry juice, cranberry leaf infusion, tea and water were used. These drinks have a slight diuretic effect and increase the sensitivity of the bladder to filling and emptying. An additional effect is the action of a natural uroseptic. After each intake of liquid, they were accustomed to going to the toilet.

The next stage of treatment is drug therapy. The presence of detrusor-sphincter dyssinergia and a shortage of blood filling of the anterior parts of the pelvis determines the appointment of alpha-blockers. We use doxazosin, tamsulosin, alfuzosin. Our patient used the drug doxazosin at a dose of 0.5 mg before bedtime. Given the likelihood of such a side effect as an orthostatic decrease in blood pressure, we give alpha-blockers when the child is already in bed and does not get up until the morning.

Taking into account the recurrent course of pyelonephritis, after the above course of antibacterial therapy, drugs from the group of uroseptics – nitrofurans (drug furagin) at a dose of 50 mg 3 times a day for 10 days and then for another 30 days only at night were prescribed. After furagin, treatment with uroseptics of plant origin continues, we use the drug "Canefron" - courses every 3 months for 3 weeks.

The next stage is combined physiotherapy treatment. The methods of physiotherapy in our patient were selected for the following actions. Low-intensity laser radiation is aimed at activating blood circulation in the pelvis. Biofeedback therapy is aimed at normalizing the group of urination reflexes that ensure the opening of the sphincter and the flow of urine [11-12]. Activation of the closing function of the uretero–vesical junction was provided by sinusoidal modulating currents in the antidystrophic mode. Physiotherapy courses were conducted every 3 months.

Against the background of the therapy for 6 months, no episodes of exacerbation of pyelonephritis were noted. With monthly monitoring of urine tests, normal results were obtained. After 6 months of treatment, a second examination was performed. The examination included performing miction cystography, uroflowmetry with pelvic floor electromyography, ultrasound examination of the urinary system and rheopelviography. The most important result was obtained during miction cystography – vesicoureteral reflux was not detected. Uroflowmetry revealed a normal type of curve – it had a domed appearance and electromyography of the pelvic floor recorded an electromyographic pause during voiding. During the rheopelviography, positive dynamics was noted in the form of normalization of blood supply to the bladder both in the filling phase and in the emptying phase. During the control ultrasound examination of the organs of the urinary system, no pathology was detected. Even the compaction of the walls of the cup-pelvic systems of the kidneys, which was revealed during the first study, was stopped.

The patient was given recommendations for continuing treatment at home. It is recommended to continue the program of behavioral therapy – drinking and urination regimen, continue courses of physiotherapy, the use of herbal uroseptics and conduct periodic monitoring of urine tests.

Conclusion. Using this clinical example, we wanted to show that the development of vesicoureteral reflux can be influenced by detrusor-sphincter dyssinergia. This is a rather dangerous violation of urodynamics, in which there is no possibility of complete relaxation of the sphincter and the flow of urine is hindered by high pressure in the urethra. Dysfunctional urination, or detrusor-sphincter dyssinergia, is manifested by prolonged emptying of the bladder with the need to strain the abdominal press, as well as periodically occurring uncontrolled abrupt interruption of urine flow. Detrusor-sphincter dyssinergia is the most common variant of functional infravesical obstruction. Unlike other variants of neurogenic bladder dysfunctions, with detrusor-sphincter dyssinergia, urinary incontinence is usually not detected and for this reason, this condition is often diagnosed only at the stage of complications, as in the described clinical observation. The main complications are vesicoureteral reflux and recurrent course of chronic pyelonephritis.

The pathogenesis of detrusor-sphincter dyssinergia is based on the following pathophysiological mechanisms. The activity of the urethral sphincter in detrusor-sphincter dyssinergia is due to a violation of the function of the miction center of the pons, which normally ensures the coordinated work of the detrusor and the external sphincter of the urethra, as well as the classical urination reflexes that ensure the emptying phase. The sequence of activation of 7-11 urination reflexes is disrupted: detrusor-urethral inhibitory, detrusor-sphincteral inhibitory, urethro-detrusor activating, urethro-sphincteral inhibitory and early activation of the 12th reflex – perineo-bulbar inhibitory. Normally, during miction, reflexes 7-11 provide a free flow of urine through the urethra by continuing the reduction of detrusor to emptying the bladder and synchronizing this reduction with relaxation of the sphincter, and the 12th reflex completes the emptying phase, activating the sphincter. The representations in the nervous system of these reflexes are different. Thus, in the detrusor-urethral inhibitory reflex, nerve centers are located in the S2-S4 segments of the spinal cord, and afferentation and efferentation are carried out along the pelvic nerves. In the detrusor-sphincteral inhibitory reflex, the nerve centers are localized in S1- S2, the afferent part of the reflex arc is the pelvic nerves, and the efferent part is the sacral nerves. There are two urethro-detrusor activating reflexes: in the 9th, the centers are located in the cranial part of the brain and in the S1-S2 segments, the afferent pathways are the lateral bundles and the sacral nerves, the efferent ones are the lateral reticulospinal tract and pelvic nerves; in the 10th reflex, the centers are the segments S2–S4, afferentation and efferentation are carried out along the pelvic nerves. In the urethro-sphincteral inhibitory reflex, the central representation is localized in the pudendal nuclei of the sacral part of the spinal cord, afferent and efferent impulses pass through the sacral nerves. The centers of the perineo-bulbar inhibitory reflex are the medulla oblongata and the sacral spinal cord. The afferent pathway is the sacrobulbar tract and the sacral nerves, the efferent pathway is the ventral reticulospinal tract [13]. As can be seen from the data presented above, the function of urination is provided by the synchronous operation of many representations in the central nervous system and by conducting pathways. Their development often goes disproportionately, a delay in the maturation of certain neuroanatomic structures may be detected. In such conditions, the uncoordinated activation of various urination reflexes is quite understandable [14].

The beginning of the act of urination is determined by an increase in the detrusor voltage at the end of the filling phase. The muscles of the anterior abdominal wall are fixed, intra-abdominal pressure increases, the pelvic floor relaxes and falls. At this point, the pressure of closing the urethra should decrease, the detrusor begins to contract and the neck of the bladder opens. With detrusor-sphincter dyssinergia, the onset of urination may be delayed due to the lack of relaxation of the urethral sphincter or with insufficient relaxation. At the same time, patients complain of difficulties at the beginning of urination. Detrusor pressure increases, when the pressure level in the urethra is exceeded, urination begins. The manifestation of detrusor hypertension during urination for a long time causes hypertrophy of the bladder muscles, the appearance of mucosal trabecularity.

In addition to difficulties at the beginning of the act of urination, patients with detrusor-sphincter dyssinergia may complain of frequent urination, the need to strain the abdominal press to urinate.

The development of complications is based on the following pathophysiological mechanisms. In conditions of obstructive urination, complete emptying is impossible, a residual volume of urine appears. When the sphincter is activated during miction, the laminar flow of urine acquires the features of a turbulent section of the urethra along the periphery, and if the flow is completely abruptly interrupted, a reversible flow of urine from the urethra to the bladder appears. In this case, infection of residual urine in the bladder occurs. Excessive detrusor pressure during miction determines a violation of the closure function of the uretero-vesical anastomosis and vesicoureteral reflux is formed. Infected urine reflux into the kidney, supporting pyelonephritis. In connection with the above information, the correct treatment of detrusor-sphincter dyssinergia makes it possible to stop vesicoureteral reflux without surgical interventions.

This study was performed using the Unique Scientific Unit (UNU) "Multicomponent software and hardware system for automated collection, storage, markup of research and clinical biomedical data, their unification and analysis based on Data Center with Artificial Intelligence technologies" (reg. number: 2075518).

References

[1] "Urinary system infections in children: A guide for doctors." Dlin V. V., Osmanov I. M., CHugunova O. L., ed. Moscow: Overlej, 2017: 262–285. (in Russ.)

[2] Morozov D. A., Morozova O. L., Mal'ceva L. D., Lakomova D. YU., Palatova T. V., Morozov D. D., Morozov K. D. "Urinary indicators of inflammation and fibrosis in children with congenital uropathies." Pediatriya im. G.N. Speranskogo. [Pediatrics named after G. N. Speransky]. 2018; 97 (5): 19–27. DOI: 10.24110/0031-403X-2018-97-5- 19-27. (in Russ.)

[3] Zajkova N. M., Dlin V. V., Karaman A., Korsunskij A. A., Eremeeva A. V., Sinicyna L. V., Revenko N. E. "The state of intrarenal hemodynamics in children with vesicoureteral reflux and reflux nephropathy." Pediatriya im. G. N.

Speranskogo. [Pediatrics named after G. N. Speransky]. 2017; 96 (5): 32–36. doi: 10.24110/0031- 403X-2017-96-5-32-36. (in Russ.)

[4] Zajkova N. M., Dlin V. V., Sinicyna L. A., Korsunskij A. A., Gackan SH. G. "Markers for determining the degree of fibrogenesis in children with vesicoureteral reflux». *Pediatriya im. G. N. Speranskogo.* [Pediatrics named after G. N. Speransky]. 2015; 94 (3): 45–51. (in Russ.)

[5] Ignatova M. S., Morozov S. L., Kryganova T. A., SHenceva D. V., Nazarova N. F., Kon'kova N. E., Dlin V. V. "Modern ideas about congenital anomalies of the organs of the urinary system (CAKUT syndrome) in children." *Klinicheskaya Nefrologiya.* [Clinical Nephrology.] 2013; 2: 58–64. (in Russ.)

[6] Kulaev A. V., Sharkov S. M. "Correction of defects of the ureterovesical segment with complete doubling of the upper urinary tract in children." *Voprosy prakticheskoj pediatrii.* [Questions of practical pediatrics.] 2021; 16 (1): 52–57. doi: 10.20953/1817-7646-2021- 1-52-57. (in Russ.)

[7] Deryugina L. A. "Vesicoureteral reflux and its prenatal prognosis." *Pediatriya im. G. N. Speranskogo.* [Pediatrics named after G. N. Speransky]. 2018; 97 (5): 14–19. DOI: 10.24110/0031-403X2018-97-5-14-19. (in Russ.)

[8] Yur'eva E. A., Dlin V. V., Vozdvizhenskaya E. S. "Genetic factors of hereditary phenotypes of vesicoureteral reflux and reflux nephropathy." *Rossijskij vestnik perinatologii i pediatrii.* [Russian Bulletin of Perinatology and Pediatrics.] 2020; 65 (3): 32–38. https://doi.org/10.21508/1027-4065-2020-65-3-32-38. (in Russ.)

[9] Pykov M. I. *"Guide. Measurements in pediatric ultrasound diagnostics».* Moscow: Publishing House "Vidar-M», 2018: 23. (in Russ.)

[10] Shahnovskij D. S., Zorkin S. N., Savost'yanov K. V., Pushkov A. A. "Genetics of vesicoureteral reflux." *Detskaya hirurgiya.* [Pediatric Surgery] 2018; 22 (4): 193–198. https://doi. org/10.18821/1560-9510-2018-22-4-193-198. (in Russ.)

[11] Guseva N. B., Nikitin S. S. "Neurophysiological aspects of urinary disorders of inorganic genesis in children, basic principles of diagnosis and treatment." *Pediatriya im. G. N. Speranskogo.* [Pediatrics named after G. N. Speransky]. 2017; 96 (5):137-144 (in Russ.)

[12] Gatkin E. YA. (ed), Guseva N.B., Hlebutina N.S. "Rehabilitation exercise therapy complexes for children with pelvic floor muscle pathology." In: *Methods of correction of neurogenic bladder dysfunction in children.* Moscow, 2022: 53–56 (in Russ.)

[13] *"Disorders of the bladder function in children and methods of urodynamic examination: a textbook for students in the areas of training of the specialty Pediatrics and General medicine."* S. S. Nikitin, N. B.Guseva. Petrozavodsk: PetrSU Publishing House, 2020. — 68 p. (in Russ.)

[14] Bozhendaev T. L., Guseva N. B., Ignat'ev R. O., Nikitin S. S. "Dysfunctional urination as a marker of neurogenic bladder disorders in children." *Pediatriya. im. G. N. Speranskogo* [Pediatrics named after G. N. Speransky].2015; 94(3):158-162. (in Russ.)

Chapter 6

Neurological Disorders and the Formation of Vesicoureteral Reflux in Children Operated on for Anorectal Malformations

Sergei Nikitin[1,2,*]**, MD**
Natalia Guseva[3,4,5]**, MD**
Svetlana Kononova[6]
and Vadim Nikitin[1]

[1]Medical institute, Petrozavodsk State University, Petrozavodsk, Russia
[2]Children's Republican Hospital named after I. N. Grigovich, Petrozavodsk, Russia
[3]Russian Medical Academy of Continuous Professional Education, Moscow, Russia
[4]Department of Pediatric Surgery, Pirogov Medical University, Moscow, Russia
[5]Moscow Voiding Dysfunction Center, Moscow Paediatric Speransky Hospital No. 9, Moscow, Russia
[6]Department of Pediatrics and Pediatric Surgery, Medical Institute of PetrSU, Petrozavodsk, Russia

Abstract

After a certain number of years after surgery for anorectal malformations, children sometimes complain of impaired urination function. The most typical complaints are manifestations of urgent urination, enuresis, difficulties at the beginning of urination and stress urinary incontinence. Such a combination of disorders is formed at an early age, it's just that operations for anorectal malformations are performed at an age when the act of urination is still unconscious and urination disorders are not detected. It is known that 45% of pelvic organ dysfunction is combined

---

[*] Corresponding Author's Email: ssnikitin@yandex.ru.

In: Vesicoureteral Reflux
Editor: Garry M. Morones
ISBN: 979-8-89113-444-7
© 2024 Nova Science Publishers, Inc.

and this applies not only to functional disorders, but also to developmental abnormalities, including anorectal malformations. Violations of pelvic functions have common mechanisms of development, which are due to the close anatomical and physiological connections of the bladder and rectum. The innervation of the muscles involved in the physiology of the act of defecation and urination is almost identical - these are sympathetic fibers of the n.hypogastricus, parasympathetic fibers of the pelvic nerves and somatic innervation – n.pudendus. The act of defecation and the act of urination are performed by similar reflex mechanisms. At the same time, the role of "detrusor" during defecation belongs to the abdominal press.

Patients and methods. For 15 years, 50 patients who had previously been operated on for anorectal malformations were examined. In all cases, surgical correction of defects was completed by the age of 18 months. At the time of the appeal, the age of the children was 4-15 years, 40 girls and 10 boys.

Manifestations of urgent urination were noted in 38 children (72%), enuresis – in 25 children (50%), difficulties at the beginning of urination – in 8 children (16%), stress urinary incontinence – in 16 children (32%). With these violations of urination, the evacuation function of the colon and rectum was quite satisfactory.

Methods of examination – assessment of clinical manifestations by the method of qualimetry of pelvic disorders, urodynamic examination, rheopelviography, miction cystography, irrigoscopy, ultrasound examination of the abdominal cavity and urinary system, laboratory urine tests.

Methods of treatment - behavioral therapy, including "urological" and "proctological" parts. From the means of drug therapy, M-hodinoblockers, alpha-blockers, periodic courses of antibacterial therapy were used. In addition, physiotherapy methods: biofeedback therapy, magnetolaser on the bladder area, acupuncture. The duration of treatment was 6 months.

After treatment, miction cystography, urodynamic examination and rheopelviography were repeated.

Results. The first degree of violations was detected in 22 children (44%), the second degree – in 18 children (36%), the third degree of violations was noted in 10 children (20%). During retrograde cystometry, hyperreflexia was revealed in all patients – a decrease in the maximum cystometric capacity by 25-55% relative to the age norm. Detrusor maladaptation was detected in 24% of children – during the filling phase, non-inhibited contractions of detrusor with a pressure from 17 to 82 cm H2O were recorded. During urethral profilometry, a decrease in urethral closure pressure (from 50 to 60 cm H2O) was determined in 16 children (32%). Rheopelviography indicators indicated a decrease in blood filling in the region.

During miction cystography, vesicoureteral reflux was detected in 22 children: in 18 children it was unilateral, in 4 children it was bilateral. The degree of reflux in 20 patients is the second, in one – the first and in another – the third. In addition, it is important that children with vesicoureteral reflux are patients with the third degree of disorders (all 10 people) and 12 children with the second degree of disorders.

Laboratory tests of urine showed the presence of an infection of the urinary system.

After a 6-month course of treatment, significant positive dynamics was noted: manifestations of neurogenic dysfunction of the bladder and vesicoureteral refluxes were stopped. At the same time, surgical treatment was not required. Conservative measures were simultaneously aimed at the treatment of violations of the act of urination and correction of evacuation function of the colon and rectum.

In conclusion, a rehabilitation program for the restoration of bladder function and conservative treatment of vesicoureteral reflux in children operated on earlier for anorectal malformations is presented.

Keywords: vesicoureteral reflux, overactive bladder, anal-rectal malformations, combined pelvic organ dysfunction, children

Introduction

Operations for anorectal malformations are performed in early childhood. At the time of the operation and in the postoperative period, the act of urination still has a conditioned reflex character and possible violations of urination do not manifest themselves. Restoration of the function of the colon and rectum with the optimal course of the postoperative period is completed in the first years of the child's life. This is the age when the act of urination has not yet been fully formed. In this regard, some of its disorders (nocturnal enuresis, urine leakage during the day, and others) are not considered as manifestations of pathology. And only a few years later it becomes clear that these manifestations are not related to the delay in the formation of the act of urination, but are a violation requiring correction.

It is known that about 45% of functional disorders of the pelvic organs (bladder and colon) are combined. With anorectal abnormalities, neurogenic bladder dysfunctions are also common. Violations of pelvic functions have common mechanisms of development, which are caused by close anatomical and physiological connections of the bladder and rectum [1].

The innervation of the muscles involved in the physiology of the act of defecation and urination is almost identical - these are sympathetic fibers of the submandibular nerve, parasympathetic fibers of the pelvic nerve and somatic innervation – the genital nerve. When the parasympathetic centers are excited in the S2-4 segments, the detrusor and longitudinal muscles of the sigmoid and rectum contract with simultaneous relaxation of their internal sphincters. When the sympathetic centers are excited in the L1-2 segments of the spinal cord, relaxation processes are detected in similar structures. At the same time, the contraction of internal sphincters is activated, which contributes to the retention of urine and feces. [2-3]. Thus, the act of defecation and the act of urination are performed by similar reflex mechanisms. At the same time, the role of "detrusor" during defecation belongs to the abdominal press.

During the act of urination, the internal sphincter of the rectum is responsible for anal retention, while the bioelectric activity of the external sphincter is absent at this time (vesico-anal reflex) [3, 4].

Normal acts of defecation and urination are impossible without synchronous contraction and relaxation of the pelvic floor. The external urethral sphincter is in a state of constant tonic activity and prevents the opening of the urethra during contraction of the m.levator ani during tension. M.levator ani contractions do not allow lowering of the neck of the bladder, while along with a sharp rise in intra-abdominal pressure, intraurethral pressure increases sharply to retain urine [3, 5].

The pelvic floor muscles regulate the function of the pelvic diaphragm and interact abdominal pressure with the urethra and anal canal. No matter how different the pathogenesis factors of combined pelvic organ dysfunction are, they are united by pelvic floor dysfunction [6]. In addition, there is also a mutual pathological mechanical effect of the bladder on the rectum and vice versa. With cholestasis, fecal stones squeeze the bladder, which leads to lymphostasis, the appearance of residual urine, incontinence or obstruction of urination, bladder dysfunction and provoke the development of vesicoureteral reflux and urinary system infection [1, 7].

Patients and Methods

Over 15 years, we have examined 50 patients who had previously been operated on for anorectal malformations. The gender distribution is as follows: 40 girls and 10 boys. Among the girls there are 32 patients - girls with anorectal atresia with recto–vestibular fistula, 2 patients with recto-vaginal fistula, 2 patients with recto-perineal fistula and 4 patients with anal canal stenosis. Among boys – 6 children with anorectal atresia without fistulas and 4 - with anorectal atresia with recto-perineal fistula. In all cases, surgical correction of defects was completed by the age of 18 months. At the time of the appeal, the age of the children was 4-15 years (4-7 years – 24 children, 8-11 years – 17 children and 12-15 years – 9 children). The reason for seeking medical help was urination disorders. Manifestations of urgent urination were noted in 38 children (72%), enuresis – in 25 children (50%), difficulties at the beginning of urination – in 8 children (16%), stress urinary incontinence – in 16 children (32%). With these violations of urination, the evacuation function of the colon and rectum was quite satisfactory. Only 10 children periodically had constipation for 3-4 days and encopresis on the fourth day of stool retention, which were corrected by performing a cleansing enema at home.

Violations of pelvic organ function are assessed by the previously developed method of qualimetry of pelvic disorders (patent No. 2472447, dated 25.08.2011). The method is an assessment of the symptoms of pelvic organ dysfunction in points, depending on the amount of which there are three degrees of violations, where the first is the lightest degree, the third is the heaviest. In this work, all children underwent the same methods of examination. But the meaning of the distribution by degrees of violations when applying the method in the practice of pediatric urologists is to use diagnostic algorithms [8].

All children underwent urodynamic studies – uroflowmetry, cystometry and urethral profilometry. When conducting uroflowmetry, in addition to standard quantitative indicators, we determine the "type of urination curve", it can be normal, functionally obstructive, obstructively interrupted, obstructively intermittent, rapid, in the form of staccato and two-stage. Cystometry and urethral profilometry are standard studies and do not require explanation in this review.

In addition, all patients underwent a rheopelviography. Rheopelviography is not a very common study in urology, let's explain its meaning. The rheography of the anterior parts of the pelvis is recorded and only two main parameters of rheography are analyzed – the systolic amplitude of the pulse wave and the maximum speed of the rapid filling period. When analyzing the rheographic curve, we use the normative indicators that we developed earlier [9-11]. The state of blood filling of organs and tissues during rheography of various regions is judged by a sufficiently large number of parameters. Only two of these indicators are suitable for rheopelviography. The systolic amplitude of the pulse wave indicates the level of blood filling in the region, and the maximum speed of the period of rapid filling indicates the tone of the arterial bed.

The rest of the studies do not require special explanations – this is an ultrasound examination of the urinary system and abdominal organs, miction cystography, and a laboratory examination of urine was also performed. Given that patients have previously been operated on for anorectal defects and a certain number of years have already passed after the operation, patients underwent irrigoscopy.

A fairly large set of measures has been used as treatment methods. Behavioral therapy has been brought to the fore. It is represented by the "urological" and "proctological" part. Urological is a drinking regimen of 150-250 ml every 2 hours from 7 a.m. to 7 p.m. with urination after each fluid intake and an additional three urinations at intervals of 20 minutes before bedtime, as well as alarm therapy. The proctological part consists in developing a reflex to defecate in the morning. In the morning on an empty stomach, the child is offered a cool drink – up to 300 ml. After that, breakfast. After breakfast – a visit to the toilet. If there is difficulty during defecation, a suppository with glycerin or micro enema is used for 5-7 minutes. In the conclusion of the article, we will explain in more detail these questions.

Among the means of drug therapy, M-cholinoblockers were used – the drug trospium chloride, alpha-adrenoblockers – the drug doxazosin, periodic courses of antibacterial therapy – cefixime and nitrofurantoin were used. In addition, physiotherapy methods: biofeedback therapy, magnetolaser on the bladder area, acupuncture. The duration of treatment was 6 months.

After treatment, miction cystography, urodynamic examination and rheopelviography were repeated.

Results

The degree of violations was determined by the method of qualimetry of pelvic function disorders. The first degree of violations was detected in 22 children (44%), the second degree – in 18 children (36%), the third degree of violations was noted in 10 children (20%). It was in patients with the third degree that periodic constipation was noted, as mentioned above.

After the course of treatment, the first degree of violations was registered in all patients. A decrease in the degree of pelvic organ dysfunction means the relief of most clinical manifestations.

The analysis of urination diaries revealed a decrease in the average effective volume of urination by 30-50% relative to the average norm and an increase in the frequency of urination – more than 8 times a day. After the course of treatment, all patients recovered the volume of urination in accordance with age standards and the frequency of urination per day began to be from 5 to 8 times.

During retrograde cystometry, hyperreflexia was revealed in all patients – a decrease in the maximum cystometric capacity by 25-55% relative to the age norm. Detrusor maladaptation was detected in 24% of children – during the filling phase, non-inhibited contractions of detrusor with a pressure from 17 to 82 cm H_2O were recorded.

After treatment, the results of retrograde cystometry underwent significant positive changes. Hyperreflexia was registered only in 4 children (8%), although even in these children the volume of the bladder increased significantly, the decrease was only 15% on average relative to the age norm. Non-inhibited detrusor contractions were stopped in 8 children (out of 12 in whom they were detected initially). In 4 children, the number and pressure of non-inhibited contractions decreased by 2 times.

During uroflowmetry before treatment, the following types of urination were detected:

- Normal -22 children (44%),
- Obstructive (functional obstruction – a shift of the maximum flow rate to the right and a decrease in the maximum flow rate of urine) -21 children (42%),
- Rapid – 5 children (10%),
- Obstructive-intermittent – 2 children (4%).

After the course of therapy, with repeated uroflowmetry, the following types of urination were identified:

- Normal – 40 children (80%),
- Obstructive (functional obstruction – a shift of the maximum flow rate to the right and a decrease in the maximum flow rate of urine – 5 children (10%),
- Rapid - 5 children (10%).

During urethral profilometry, a decrease in urethral closure pressure (from 50 to 60 cm H_2O) was determined in 16 children (32%) – these are children who complained of stress urinary incontinence. In the remaining patients, urethral profilometry showed a normal result.

After the course of treatment, normal urethral closure pressure was determined in 10 patients, in 6 patients the urethral closure pressure increased to 65-72 cm H_2O.

During rheopelviography, the systolic amplitude of the pulse wave before treatment was 0.017 ± 0.008 Om ($M \pm \sigma$), the maximum speed of the rapid filling period was 0.22 ± 0.061 Om/sec ($M \pm \sigma$). These indicators indicate a decrease in blood supply in the region. After treatment, the systolic pulse wave amplitude was 0.028 ± 0.007 Om ($M \pm \sigma$), the maximum speed of the rapid filling period was 0.38 ± 0.021 Om/sec ($M \pm \sigma$). Thus, a significant increase in the level of microcirculation of the anterior parts of the pelvis was revealed against the background of the therapy.

Ultrasound examination of the organs of the urinary system and abdominal cavity did not provide any special information that could change tactics. In 12 children, minimal pyelectasia was detected – anterior-posterior diameter of the kidney pelvis was 10-12 mm.

Important information was obtained during miction cystography. Vesicoureteral reflux was detected in 22 children: 18 children had unilateral reflux, 4 children had bilateral reflux. The degree of reflux in 20 patients is the second, in one – the first and in another – the third. In addition, it is important that children with vesicoureteral reflux are patients with the third degree of disorders (all 10 people) and 12 children with the second degree of disorders.

Children with vesicoureteral reflux received the same conservative therapy as all other patients. None of the patients underwent endoscopic reflux correction. After treatment, during repeated miction cystography, vesicoureteral reflux was not recorded.

Laboratory tests of urine showed the presence of a secondary infection of the urinary system in all patients. Leukocyturia was detected (up to 10 in the field of vision in 28 children, 10-20 in the field of vision in 12 children and over 20 in the field of vision in 10 children).

After the course of therapy, normalization of urine tests was noted.

According to irrigoscopy, the volume of the colon in children aged 4-7 years was 1335 ± 215 ml ($M \pm \sigma$), 8-11 years – 1400 ± 212.8 ml ($M \pm \sigma$), 12-15 years – 1541.3 ± 187.6 ml ($M \pm \sigma$). In relation to the standard size of the volume for each age, the increase in the intestine was: at the age of 4-7 years – by an average of 45%, 8-11 years – by 23%, and at 12-15 years – by 40%.

The constant in the group of children aged 4-7 years was 28 ± 4.25 (M ± σ), 8-11 years – 28.2 ± 3.23 (M ± σ), 12-15 years – 30.26 ± 3.27 (M ± σ). The rectal diameter in the group of children aged 4-7 years was 4.3 ± 1.2 (M ± σ), 8-11 years – 3.8 ± 0.6 (M ± σ), 12-15 years – 4.25 ± 0.54 (M ± σ). Only the volume of the colon goes beyond the normative limits. The constant and the diameter of the rectum in operated patients are at the upper limit of the norm.

Discussion

Combined disorders of the pelvic organs represent a major social problem for children and their parents. Manifestations of violations are very annoying in a social and ethical sense symptoms that dramatically worsen the quality of life of patients and their environment. Emerging problems disrupt the social adaptation of children in society and lead to the development of psychological problems up to personality disorders [12-13].

In addition to the violation of the quality of life in the presence of symptoms of pelvic organ dysfunction, the formation of complications is important. Among the complications, the most common are urinary system infection and vesicoureteral reflux. It is known that these complications over time can lead to the development of chronic renal failure. Therefore, it is necessary to treat this category of patients without waiting for the independent resolution of symptoms of pelvic organ dysfunction with age.

The results of all the survey methods obtained are interdependent. The higher the degree of pelvic organ dysfunction, the greater the likelihood of the formation of vesicoureteral reflux.

Normalization of pelvic organ function with a decrease in clinical manifestations and a decrease in the degree of pelvic organ dysfunction occurs when microcirculation is activated in the projection of the pelvis. To study regional blood circulation, there are two main methods - ultrasound Dopplerography and rheography. Ultrasound Dopplerography is limited by the anatomical features of the region - the availability of vessels for location and their diameter. Rheography allows you to solve the problem with the help of rheopelviography. Considering that the sympathetic department of the autonomic nervous system is responsible for tissue perfusion, the results obtained suggest the presence of its increased activity in this category of patients, which is one of the pathogenetic moments in the development of pelvic organ dysfunction. This fact makes it possible to prescribe pathogenetically justified treatment with alpha-blockers. An increase in the systolic amplitude of the pulse wave and the maximum speed of the rapid filling period after treatment with an alpha-adrenoblocker show activation of blood flow to the region and restoration of pelvic organ function. Clinical manifestations of the disease began to decrease in parallel with the activation of pelvic blood flow. The dependence of the sum of points (calculated by the method of qualimetry) is revealed from the indicators of the rheopelviographic study. The better the blood filling of tissues, the less clinical manifestations of the disease. There was an increase in the average effective volume of urination, and the number of urinations per day, respectively, decreased to standard values. In addition, urodynamic parameters have significantly improved: the maximum cystometric capacity has increased. In most children, non-inhibited contractions were stopped, and in the observations where they continued to be detected, the number and pressure of non-inhibited detrusor contractions decreased. Against the background of the therapy, uroflowmetric indicators also underwent pronounced positive dynamics. Pathological types of urination – obstructive-intermittent and rapid - have ceased to be determined. Most urination after treatment is of the normal type, in other cases there was a small functional obstruction, which was expressed in the form of a shift of the peak of the maximum flow rate of urine to the right and a slight decrease in the maximum flow rate of urine.

Improvement of blood circulation and the associated activation of the energy metabolism of the detrusor and colon are likely links in the process that led to positive changes in the reservoir function of the pelvic organs. The reason for the improvement of hemodynamics of the pelvic organs was the blockade of alpha-adrenoreceptors of the vessels of the colon and bladder, which eliminated vascular spasm and manifestations of pelvic ischemia.

The bladder and colon are in close anatomical and functional connection due to the common mechanisms of innervation, blood supply and similar embryonic origin. They perform the same type of tasks (accumulation and evacuation), which are provided by the function of the pelvic floor muscles [14-15]. Violation of the productivity of the evacuation function of the colon is manifested by the presence of constipation, sometimes with secondary encopresis, and an increase in the volume of the colon. Overactive bladder, on the contrary, is characterized by imperative urination syndrome (urgency), manifested by frequent urination, small effective volumes of the bladder and imperative urges with or without urinary incontinence. That is, the phenomena, in principle, are the opposite of each other – "stretching" of the intestine and a decrease in the volume of the bladder. But it turns out that there is a relationship between these phenomena. It can be argued that these phenomena have a single pathogenetic basis, which is associated with the activity of the sympathetic department of the autonomic nervous system. Activation of alpha-adrenergic receptors is manifested initially by spasm, and with prolonged exposure - by hypoxia, which further causes secondary changes in the neuromuscular structures of the rectum and bladder [16-17]. Thus, the main pathogenetic link in the development of combined pelvic disorders is a lesion at the level of the microcirculatory bed. Activation of blood circulation with restoration of pelvic functions made it possible to restore the closure function of the uretero-vesical anastomosis and to stop vesicoureteral reflux.

Conclusion

In conclusion, it should be noted the need to control not only the evacuation function of the colon and rectum in patients operated on for anorectal malforrnations, but also the function of the bladder. General functions, blood supply systems and innervation determine the combination of these disorders. Neurogenic disorders of urination in children operated on for anorectal defects are clearly manifested several years after surgery and the significance of symptoms in terms of reducing the quality of life comes to the fore. These disorders are complicated by infection of the urinary system and the formation of vesicoureteral reflux.

It is likely that it is necessary to find out the presence of urinary dysfunction in children operated on for anorectal abnormalities as early as possible for timely correction and prevention of complications. It is even more correct to draw up a rehabilitation program immediately after the child's discharge from the hospital after surgery for anorectal anomaly, taking into account the control of bladder function. The purpose of this program is to minimize or completely exclude clinical manifestations of pelvic organ dysfunction and the associated normal growth, development and, in the future, social adaptation of the child in society, the opportunity to study at a comprehensive school or attend a preschool together with healthy children, as well as to prevent the development of complications of the disease. The implementation of this program is a very painstaking event and requires close attention and diligence from parents and adults around the child, but only its clear execution can guarantee a successful result.

Teaching parents or guardians and patients to change their usual lifestyle, to form a responsible attitude to the problem from an early age is aimed at obtaining a high degree of control over the function of the pelvic organs. This includes proper hydration regimens, forced urination and defecation.

The correct hydration regimen is, in most cases, the starting point for stabilizing the physiological rhythm of urination and defecation. The regimen and control of the age-related volume of fluid consumed is prescribed by the doctor to the patient for a period of at least three months. Physiological fluid intake is calculated taking into account the weight of the child, and, depending on age, in children 1-15 years old, is 50-120 ml / kg / day [18]. The daily intake of liquid is distributed evenly during the first ten hours of wakefulness, every 2 hours and, necessarily, a glass of water at room temperature immediately after waking up.

Due to the slowdown in the formation of the age-related cortical rhythm of patients, parents or guardians need to monitor the correctness of the doctor's recommendations. Approximately from 4-5 years of age, an individual control regime is prescribed when a parent or guardian does not control the drinking regimen and urination regimen of the child once every three weeks during the day, checking the degree of formation of the child's responsibility in the implementation of routine medical recommendations – independent regular fluid intake in a given volume.

In combination with working out the hydration regimen, given the protracted process of becoming a mature type of urination, compliance with the regimen of forced urination is required for patients under the supervision of parents or guardians. It is recommended to urinate every 2-3 hours during the day. If enuresis is present among the clinical manifestations, then the child is additionally offered to visit the toilet for an hour before going to bed three times with an interval of 20 minutes. During a night's sleep, alarm therapy can be used with the help of special devices according to the standard method from 1 to 6 months.

Children with a delay or violation of the formation of a mature type of urination should pay special attention to the observance of the daily routine. The child should not be overloaded with various activities during the day, then the depth threshold of his night sleep will correspond to the possibility of disinhibition, if necessary, to respond to signals from the external and internal environment, including the emerging urge to urinate. For the same purpose, it is even recommended to give the child the opportunity to have a nap, regardless of age, for at least 1-2 hours.

Daily adequate bowel emptying usually prevents the occurrence of episodes of secondary encopresis. Its appearance during daily emptying may indicate incomplete emptying during defecation. Encopresis in the first years after surgery for anorectal malformations can sometimes appear during the day, as the rectum is filled with contents, even in the case of complete bowel emptying in the morning. This is usually due to insufficiency of the external sphincter of the rectum. In this situation, the defecation mode is selected depending on the time during which the child can be clean after another defecation. A prerequisite is periodic courses of treatment aimed at stimulating the anal sphincter – sinusoidal modulating currents on the perineum, massage, physical therapy, biofeedback therapy, regular courses of training enemas. Training enemas are recommended to be performed in the evening. A small volume of liquid (boiled water at room temperature) is injected shallowly into the rectum and the child is asked to hold this water as long as possible, physical activity is encouraged during retention. Thus, the external sphincter of the rectum is "trained." Note the retention time and, when it increases, increase the amount of injected liquid (for example, from 50 to 100-150 ml).

Children with combined pelvic organ dysfunction should be taught hygiene skills from an early age, explaining the danger of ascending urinary infection.

An important component of the rehabilitation program is regular visits to a specialist with condition monitoring by qualimetry and timely correction of therapy according to indications.

This study was performed using the Unique Scientific Unit (UNU) «Multicomponent software and hardware system for automated collection, storage, markup of research and clinical biomedical data, their unification and analysis based on Data Center with Artificial Intelligence technologies» (reg. number: 2075518).

References

[1] Kol'be O. B., Sazonov A. N., Moiseev A. B., Larina L. E., Petrosova S. A., Labutina N. V., Badyaeva S. A. "Combined disorders of the function of the bladder and colon in children." *Pediatriya*. 2003;6:1-4 (in Russ.).

[2] Filin V. A., Petrosova S. A., Alieva E. I., Kol'be O. B., Poddubnyj I. V., Fajzulin A. K. "Etiopathogenetic aspects of combined disorders of the function of the bladder and distal colon in children." *Pediatriya*. 2006;5:97-99. (in Russ.).

[3] Hachatryan V. A., Orlov Yu. A., Osipov I. B., Elikbaev G. M. "Spinal dysraphy: neurosurgical and neurological aspects." Saint-Petersburg: "*Desyatka*", 2009: 304. (in Russ.).

[4] Berlej D. E., Melo A. D. "Coloproctology and pelvic floor. Pathophysiology and treatment." ed. M. M. Henry, M. Svosh; translated from English by N. B. Morozov, V.L.Rivkin. Moscow: "Medicina", 1998: 464. (in Russ.).

[5] Salov P. P. *"Neurogenic dysfunction of the pelvic organs."* Novokuznetsk, 2002: 592. (in Russ.).

[6] Ivanovskij Yu. V., Smirnov M. A. "Morphofunctional justifications for the use of the biofeedback method in urology and proctology." *Posobie dlya vrachej.* Saint-Petersburg. 2003: 21. (in Russ.).

[7] Nordling J., Meyhoff, H. H. "Dissotiation of urethral and anal sphincter activity in neurogenic bladder dysfunction." *J. Urol.* 1979;122(3):352-356.

[8] Nikitin S. S. "Combined pelvic organ dysfunction in children." *Medicinskij akademicheskij zhurnal.* 2011; 1:75-80 (in Russ.).

[9] Romashin M. A., Guseva N. B., Nikitin S. S., Gatkin E. Ya. "The relevance of studying the state of blood circulation of the bladder in children with its neurogenic disorders." *Medicinskij sovet.* 2023;17(1):118–122. (in Russ.) https://doi.org/10.21518/ms2022-014.

[10] Nikitin S. S., Grigovich I. N., Elagina R. A., Syutina A. V., Toksubaeva E. P. "Reographical studies of pelvic blood flow in the diagnosis of pelvic organ dysfunction in children." Vestnik eksperimental'noj i klinicheskoj hirurgii. *Nauchno-prakticheskij zhurnal.* Prilozhenie. [Bulletin of experimental and clinical surgery. Scientific and practical journal. Application] 2011: 41-43 (in Russ.).

[11] Nikitin S. S., Elagina R. A., Syutina A. V., Toksubaeva E. P. *"Diagnosis of pelvic blood flow disorders by rheopelviography in children."* Petrozavodskie pediatricheskie chteniya – VII: fiziologiya i patologiya detskogo vozrasta: [Petrozavodsk pediatric readings - VII: physiology and pathology of childhood]: Materials of the scientific and practical conference (Petrozavodsk, May 21-22, 2010). Petrozavodsk: Publishing House of PetrSU, 2010:70-71(in Russ.).

[12] Ignat'ev R. O., Guseva N. B., Nikitin S. S., Ryzhov E. A., Fomenko O. Yu., Ponomareva T. N. "Opportunities to improve the quality of life of children with combined urination and defecation disorders with the unification of diagnostic and treatment methods." *Detskaya hirurgiya.* 2014;5:8-12(in Russ.).

[13] Malyh A. L. "Modern features of diagnosis and treatment of disorders of visceral organs in children and adolescents with neurogenic dysfunction of the bladder and colon." *Medicinskij al'manah.* 2010; 3(12):156-160 (in Russ.).

[14] Vishnevskij E. L., Guseva N. B. "Justification of treatment of neurogenic bladder in children with picamilon." *Urologiya i nefrologiya.* 1998;2:27-30. (in Russ.).

[15] Buyanov M. I. "Urinary and fecal incontinence." Moscow: *"Medicina"*, 1985:184 c. (in Russ.).

[16] Berezhanskaya T. I., Nikitin S. S. "Treatment of patients with a combination of vesicoureteral reflux and neurogenic bladder dysfunction." Materials of the II Russian Congress "Modern Technologies in Pediatrics and Pediatric Surgery." Moscow: *"Medpraktika"*, 2003: 452. (in Russ.).

[17] Lenyushkin A. I., Kim L. A., Ryzhov E. A., Tsapkin A. E. "Evolution of the view on the etiopathogenesis of chronic constipation in children." *Detskaya hirurgiya.* 2009;6:48-50. (in Russ.).

[18] Husu E. P., Nikitin S. S., Rianov V. V., Tarasov S. V. "Infusion therapy in children with surgical diseases." *Uchebnoe posobie*. Ed. I. N. Grigovich. Petrozavodsk: Publishing House of Petr SU, 2013:66. (in Russ.).

Index

A

acute kidney injury (AKI), 2, 7, 10, 12, 13, 18, 19, 23, 25, 30
American Urological Association (AUA), 17, 19, 30
anal-rectal malformations, 97
apoptotic bodies, 4, 6
aquaporin 2 (AQP2), 6, 10, 11
atonic bladder, 53, 61

B

biofluids, 7, 17
biogenesis, 4, 6
biomarkers, vii, 1, 2, 3, 7, 8, 9, 10, 11, 12, 13, 16, 17, 18, 19, 21, 22, 23, 24, 25, 26, 28, 29, 30, 31
bladder, vii, 1, 3, 6, 7, 12, 13, 14, 16, 28, 34, 35, 37, 38, 40, 41, 42, 43, 45, 46, 47, 48, 49, 51, 52, 54, 55, 56, 57, 58, 59, 60, 61, 62, 63, 64, 65, 68, 69, 70, 71, 72, 73, 74, 76, 77, 78, 79, 80, 83, 84, 85, 87, 88, 89, 90, 91, 92, 93, 96, 97, 98, 100, 101,104, 105, 107, 108
bulking agents, 19

C

cell-to-cell communication, 7
chemokine, 20, 30
children, vii, 3, 4, 15, 17, 18, 22, 25, 29, 30, 31, 33, 34, 35, 39, 40, 41, 42, 44, 45, 46, 47, 48, 49, 51, 53, 54, 57, 60, 63, 64, 65, 67, 68, 69, 71, 74, 78, 79, 80, 81, 85, 86, 92, 93, 95, 96, 97, 99, 100, 101, 102, 103, 104, 105, 106, 107, 108, 109
chronic kidney disease (CKD), 7, 10, 12, 14, 18, 23, 25, 27, 30, 56, 68, 69
combined dysfunction of the pelvic organs, 37, 68, 79, 80
combined pelvic organ dysfunction, vii, 64, 68, 69, 71, 75, 78, 97, 98, 107, 108
constipation, vii, 54, 57, 62, 68, 69, 74, 75, 77, 78, 99, 100, 104, 108
cyclic VCUG, 4, 18
cystourethrography, 1, 3, 15, 18, 19, 20, 21, 22, 30

D

Detrusor-sphincter dyssinergia, 55, 84, 85, 88, 89, 90, 91, 92
diagnosis, 3, 7, 17, 18, 21, 26, 35, 36, 37, 38, 39, 40, 48, 49, 53, 57, 64, 67, 75, 77, 78, 79, 80, 86, 88, 93, 108
diagnostic(s), vii, 1, 2, 10, 17, 18, 21, 23, 24, 26, 33, 39, 40, 48, 57, 79, 84, 88, 93, 99, 108
disease(s), 1, 2, 3, 7, 9, 10, 11, 12, 14, 18, 21, 22, 23, 24, 25, 26, 27, 28, 29, 30, 31, 36, 37, 41, 42, 47, 60, 84, 86, 104, 105, 109
drug delivery, 3, 7, 12, 22, 24, 27
dysfunction, 14, 33, 34, 35, 37, 40, 48, 49, 51, 52, 53, 54, 56, 58, 64, 67, 68, 69, 70, 71, 74, 77, 78, 79, 80, 83, 85, 88, 89, 93, 95, 97, 98, 99, 100, 103, 105, 108

Index

E

endoscopic injection, 19
exosomes, 3, 4, 6, 7, 12, 13, 16, 21, 22, 24, 25, 26, 27, 28
extracellular vesicles (EVs), 1, 2, 3, 4, 6, 7, 8, 9, 10, 12, 13, 16, 17, 18, 19, 21, 22, 23, 24, 25, 26, 27, 28

F

fibroblast growth factor (FGF), 15, 25
fibrosis, 2, 7, 8, 9, 15, 16, 18, 20, 25, 26, 28, 30, 92

G

genetic(s), 2, 17, 93
glomerulonephritis, 7, 10, 12, 26

I

IL-10, IL-6, IL-8, 15
inflammation, 2, 7, 15, 16, 28, 34, 37, 84, 87, 88, 92
inflammatory responses, 6
intercellular messengers, 7, 23
intermittent VUR, 4, 18
International Society of Extracellular Vesicles (ISEV), 17
intra-nephron communication, 6
invasive, 1, 2, 3, 12, 18, 19, 21, 26, 74, 78, 84, 88

K

kidney damage, vii, 1, 2, 3, 4, 7, 13, 17, 18, 37, 83, 85
kidney disease improving global outcomes (KDIGO), 12, 25
kidney transplantation (KT), 16, 20, 31, 63
kidney(s), vii, 1, 2, 3, 4, 6, 7, 10, 12, 13, 14, 15, 16, 18, 20, 21, 23, 25, 26, 27, 28, 29, 30, 31, 34, 35, 36, 37, 38, 40, 47, 49, 52, 54, 55, 56, 59, 60, 62, 63, 64, 83, 85, 87, 88, 90, 92, 102

M

malformation(s), vii, 18, 35, 38, 47, 51, 53, 54, 86, 95, 96, 97, 98, 107
microvesicles, 4, 6, 27, 28
miRNAs, 8, 13, 26

N

nephron, 6
neurogenic detrusor overactivity, 53, 58, 59

O

obstruction, 13, 14, 19, 28, 29, 37, 38, 46, 54, 55, 58, 85, 90, 98, 101, 104
organ(s), 12, 37, 42, 49, 52, 53, 62, 63, 64, 67, 68, 69, 71, 74, 75, 76, 77, 78, 79, 80, 81, 83, 85, 87, 90, 93, 95, 97, 99, 100, 102, 103, 104, 105, 106, 108
overactive bladder, 34, 35, 41, 42, 48, 49, 64, 68, 72, 75, 76, 77, 79, 80, 87, 97, 104

P

pathogenesis, 14, 25, 85, 90, 98
pathophysiology, 14, 108
patient(s), vii, 1, 2, 4, 14, 15, 16, 17, 18, 19, 20, 22, 24, 25, 26, 27, 28, 29, 30, 33, 34, 37, 39, 40, 41, 45, 46, 52, 53, 54, 55, 56, 57, 58, 59, 60, 61, 62, 63, 64, 68, 69, 74, 78, 84, 85, 88, 89, 90, 91, 92, 96, 97, 98, 99, 100, 101, 102, 103, 105, 106, 108
pediatric, 2, 4, 18, 22, 25, 31, 33, 35, 47, 48, 49, 51, 57, 64, 67, 79, 80, 81, 83, 86, 93, 95, 99, 108
pelvic, 40, 41, 42, 49, 52, 53, 54, 56, 58, 59, 61, 62, 63, 64, 67, 68, 69, 70, 71, 74, 75, 77, 78, 79, 80, 81, 84, 87, 88, 90, 91, 93, 95, 96, 97, 98, 99, 100, 103, 104, 105, 106, 108
physiological, 2, 4, 21, 38, 40, 41, 70, 77, 96, 97, 106

Index

podocyte, 7, 27
post-surgical monitoring, 19
primary VUR, 14, 17, 19
prognosis, 4, 17, 48, 79, 93
prostate, 6, 10, 11, 12, 25, 26
proteomes, 4, 7, 26
pyelonephritis, 15, 19, 33, 34, 37, 41, 47, 52, 54, 55, 57, 59, 70, 77, 83, 84, 85, 86, 87, 88, 89, 90, 92

R

reflux nephropathy, 2, 15, 34, 35, 37, 38, 45, 69, 83, 85, 92, 93
renal scars, 15, 18
RNA, 9, 10, 25

S

secondary VUR, 14
sphincter, 55, 84, 85, 88, 89, 90, 91, 92
spinal hernia, 51, 53, 54
spinal neurogenic bladder, vii, 51, 52, 53, 55, 57, 63
stem cells, 3, 12, 22, 27, 28
surgical ureteral reimplantation, 19

T

therapeutic, 3, 12, 13, 19, 22, 23, 24, 27, 28, 58, 62, 64
transforming growth factor (TGF), 8, 15, 65
transforming growth factor-β1 (TGF-β1), 8, 15, 65
treatment(s), vii, 3, 4, 17, 18, 19, 23, 27, 28, 29, 31, 33, 34, 35, 37, 40, 41, 42, 43, 45, 46, 47, 48, 49, 52, 53, 55, 56, 57, 58, 59, 60, 61, 62, 63, 64, 67, 68, 70, 71, 72, 73, 74, 75, 77, 78, 79, 80, 83, 84, 85, 86, 89, 90, 92, 93, 96, 97, 100, 101, 102, 103, 107, 108
tubular regeneration, 6
tumor, 15
tumor necrosis factor (TNF), 15
tumor necrosis factor-α (TNF-α), 15

U

underactive bladder, 53, 56, 69
urinary creatinine, 19
urinary extracellular vesicles (uEVs), vii, 1, 2, 3, 4, 6, 7, 8, 12, 14, 16, 17, 18, 19, 20, 21, 23, 26, 28
urinary Neutrophil gelatinase-associated lipocalin (uNGAL), 2, 18, 19, 30
urinary tract, vii, 1, 2, 3, 4, 14, 18, 19, 21, 22, 29, 34, 35, 36, 37, 39, 40, 41, 45, 46, 54, 55, 56, 61, 63, 64, 67, 68, 69, 70, 71, 74, 75, 78, 84, 85, 93
urinary tract infection(s), 2, 3, 22, 34, 39, 45, 68, 69, 70, 74
urodynamics, 40, 47, 53, 54, 55, 64, 88, 90

V

vascular endothelial growth factor (VEGF), 15
vesicoureteral junction (VUJ), 14, 29
vesicoureteral reflux (VUR), vii, 1, 2, 3, 4, 8, 13, 14, 15, 16, 17, 18, 19, 20, 21, 22, 23, 29, 30, 31, 33, 34, 35, 36, 37, 38, 39, 40, 41, 42, 44, 45, 46, 47, 48, 49, 51, 52, 53, 54, 57, 58, 59, 60, 61, 63, 67, 68, 69, 70, 72, 73, 74, 75, 76, 77, 78, 79, 80, 81, 83, 84, 85, 87, 88, 89, 90, 92, 93, 95, 97, 98, 102, 103, 105, 108
vitronectin, 2, 16, 21, 30
voiding, 1, 3, 15, 18, 19, 20, 21, 22, 30
voiding cystourethrography (VCUG), 1, 3, 15, 18, 19, 20, 21, 22, 30